The Last Best Cure

The Last Best Cure

*My Quest to Awaken the
Healing Parts of My Brain
and Get Back My Body,
My Joy, and My Life*

Donna Jackson Nakazawa

HUDSON
STREET
PRESS

HUDSON STREET PRESS
Published by Penguin Group
Penguin Group (USA) Inc., 375 Hudson Street, New York, New York 10014, USA •
Penguin Group (Canada), 90 Eglinton Avenue East, Suite 700, Toronto, Ontario M4P 2Y3,
Canada (a division of Pearson Penguin Canada Inc.) • Penguin Books Ltd, 80 Strand, London WC2R 0RL, England • Penguin Ireland, 25 St Stephen's Green, Dublin 2, Ireland (a
division of Penguin Books Ltd) • Penguin Group (Australia), 707 Collins Street, Mel-
bourne, Victoria 3008, Australia (a division of Pearson Australia Group Pty Ltd) •
Penguin Books India Pvt Ltd, 11 Community Centre, Panchsheel Park, New Delhi – 110
017, India • Penguin Group (NZ), 67 Apollo Drive, Rosedale, Auckland 0632, New Zealand (a division of Pearson New Zealand Ltd) • Penguin Books, Rosebank Office Park, 181
Jan Smuts Avenue, Parktown North 2193, South Africa • Penguin China, B7 Jaiming Center, 27 East Third Ring Road North, Chaoyang District, Beijing 100020, China

Penguin Books Ltd., Registered Offices: 80 Strand, London WC2R 0RL, England

First published by Hudson Street Press, a member of Penguin Group (USA) Inc.

First Printing, March 2013
10 9 8 7 6 5 4 3 2 1

REGISTERED TRADEMARK—MARCA REGISTRADA

HUDSON
STREET
PRESS

LIBRARY OF CONGRESS CATALOGING-IN-PUBLICATION DATA

Nakazawa, Donna Jackson.
  The last best cure : my quest to awaken the healing parts of my brain—and get back my
body, my joy, and my life / Donna Jackson Nakazawa.
    p. cm.
  Includes bibliographical references and index.
  ISBN 978-1-59463-128-3 (hc.)
  1. Nakazawa, Donna Jackson—Health. 2. Autoimmune diseases–Patients—United
States—Biography. 3. Autoimmune diseases—Alternative treatment. 4. Autoimmune
diseases—Psychosomatic aspects. 5. Mind and body therapies. I. Title.
  RC600.N36 2013
  616.97'80092—dc23
  [B]   2012018972

Printed in the United States of America
Set in Janson Text
Designed by Victoria Hartman

PUBLISHER'S NOTE
While the author has made every effort to provide accurate telephone numbers, Internet
addresses, and other contact information at the time of publication, neither the publisher nor
the author assumes any responsibility for errors, or for changes that occur after publication.
Further, publisher does not have any control over and does not assume any responsibility for
author or third-party Web sites or their content.

For my father

Contents

Introduction

This book began with my own sudden lockdown into the world of the chronically ill a little more than a decade ago. One day in 2001 I was pulling my daughter in a red wagon to the neighborhood pool to swim my evening mile in the lap lane. The next day I was paralyzed, unable to use my arms or legs, in Johns Hopkins Hospital with Guillain-Barré syndrome (GBS), a disease similar to multiple sclerosis but with more sudden onset and a wider array of possible outcomes.

I slowly regained my ability to walk, drive, and tie my children's shoes only to fall paralyzed with GBS again in 2005. The second recovery was harder, more tenuous. Although with miracle drugs and half a year of grueling physical therapy I could get down the steps and to my mailbox again, I still dealt with the neurological fallout of having had GBS twice—numb feet and hands, muscle spasms, poor reflexes, and a flu-like lethargy that no amount of sleep could cure.

Over the years other diagnoses unrelated to GBS had also thickened my chart: thyroiditis, more nerve damage, a clotting disorder, low red and white blood cell counts, bowel problems, slipped disks, and fevers of unknown origin. Every few months I'd end up back in crisis mode.

My team of specialists—some of the best on the planet—pulled miracles out of thin air for me time and again. A pacemaker made my heart tick, and a small, white pill kicked my thyroid into action each morning. Infusions of other peoples' healthy immune fighter proteins, or antibodies—pooled from a thousand donors in a product known as immunoglobulin—replaced my faulty ones and kept them from turning against me.

The pattern was familiar: I would recover enough to drive, cook dinner, type stories on my computer again. And for that I felt lucky. But in the span of a decade I'd gone from being a healthy working mom who could swim sixty laps and stay up until two a.m. decorating a toddler's birthday cake to being a revolving-door hospital patient— perpetually worried, exhausted, and often in pain.

Above everything, I longed for a normal, ordinary life: to play hide and seek or jump in the ocean waves with my kids again, to go for a brisk morning swim with my husband.

My team of specialists had pulled off miracle after miracle to keep me alive, but there was one cure they couldn't offer me: they couldn't give me back my capacity for joy. I felt robbed of joy.

And there was no Rx for that.

Something had been taken from me, and I wanted it back.

MEANWHILE, THE MOMENTS of everyday life that mattered most were spinning past. Life seemed to be increasing its speed while my own energy sputtered out. My best years with my children were almost behind me. My son was already in high school, my daughter nearly a teen. Soon, they would be gone. These were supposed to be my most productive and creative work years. And yet I was too tired and often in too much pain to enjoy, keep up with it all, drink it in. I was stuck not only in my body, I felt stuck in place, held back from the full life I'd always thought I'd create for myself, for my family. It was starting to be too late to hope I'd ever have more than a half-life. A maybe life.

• • •

THIS BOOK WAS born out of that personal frustration. As a science journalist I did what I often do: searched for research trends that might give me insight as to how to solve the puzzle of my own life. For years, I'd been intrigued by the growing number of studies examining how our brain's mental activity impacts our biology and well-being. But little of the science seemed geared to those facing chronic pain, discomfort, or illness.

Suddenly, however, the research had taken a quantum leap. Neurobiologists at the best research institutes in the world were finding myriad ways to peer inside the body and demonstrate how specific practices could activate robust healing responses in the brain, not only making us feel better but creating lasting biological changes in our physical body and cells.

One area of mind-body medicine intrigued me in particular: the relatively new and burgeoning field called psychoneuroimmunology, or PNI.

Psychoneuroimmunology is the study of the potent interaction between our psychological state of mind and our cellular and immune function. It examines the direct influence that states of mind—ranging from contentedness and well-being to joy and delight—have on the messages our brain sends to our immune system, our nerves, and our cells.

In simplest terms, the science of PNI—or what I have heard a few scientists call for simplicity's sake, PIN, or psycho-immu-neurology— is the study of how our mental and emotional state, the very way we think and act, can maximize our ability to heal—and enhance our overall physical health.

Their findings were giving new credence to the idea that the mind-body connection plays a critical and even determining role in our physical condition. Moreover, research was beginning to focus specifically on helping patients with chronic conditions to relieve emotional and physical pain and suffering.

Emerging data was showing that those with chronic conditions who practiced specific mind-body approaches were able to move their emotional state away from anxiety and pain—and toward more joy and well-being. In the process, their levels of inflammatory biomarkers and stress hormones—those linked to a range of diseases including fibromyalgia, digestive illnesses, Alzheimer's, autoimmune disease, depression, chronic pain, and cancer—profoundly decreased. They felt and did better.

This feedback loop made sense. You engaged in practices that helped to redirect your mental state away from anxiety, fear, and pain and toward contentment and joy. As a result, your inflammatory and stress biomarkers went down. As your mental state shifted, you felt some sense of physical relief. You *felt* you were somehow healthier. And, I imagined, if your levels of inflammation decreased, you *were* improving your physical health. No doubt, too, feeling any physical relief would help you to more easily move your mindset away from anxiety and pain, and ensure that you were more easily able to reenter that state of joy and well-being.

I felt certain it would for me.

I immediately saw how the science of PIN offers striking hope for those of us who long for a more pain-free existence. If feeling more joy and well-being and feeling better physically are so deeply and inextricably linked, then we owe it to ourselves to seek out strategies to improve our emotional state and maximize our brain's own healing response. We owe it to ourselves to reclaim joy and reengage with the fullness of life and set that feedback loop in motion. I couldn't wait to find out more.

I began by delving into stacks of peer-reviewed studies from the National Library of Medicine, reviewing recent talks given at major research conferences, and talking to the cutting-edge researchers in the field from Johns Hopkins to Emory to the National Institutes of Health to the University of California. Books began to pile up on my bedside table, including the research and writings of Daniel Amen, Tal Ben-Shahar, Ed Diener, Norman Doidge, Barbara Ehrenreich, Barbara Fredrickson, Daniel Gilbert, Jerome Groopman, Rick Hanson, Jon Kabat-Zinn, Eric Kandel, and Esther Sternberg.

The more I investigated how this connection works, the more excited I became.

PIN RESEARCHERS HAVE found that specific brain-body approaches such as meditation, mindfulness, yoga, laughter yoga, specific breathing patterns, immersion in nature, and acupuncture, among others, activate connections in our brain that can induce a mindset of joy and contentment. Accessing this enhanced state of joy and well-being significantly alters activity in our brain, which shifts our immune responses, hormone markers, and levels of various inflammatory chemicals and messenger molecules that the brain uses to send information forth to the body.

When we are stressed, worried, or in pain, this complex network of biological messengers—what scientists sometimes refer to as the "floating brain"—increases the cascade of chemical messengers that break down our cells and corrupt our immune responses. When we move to a state of joy and contentment, we create quite the opposite effect: a seemingly invisible shield of positive "floating brain" activity that protects our cells, our immune function, and our health.

Depending on our state of mind, we trigger a positive floating brain or a negative one. Joy and feelings of well-being can protect our immune systems, and lack of joy and well-being can tax our bodies and deprive our cells.

For a moment the research suddenly seemed, on a personal level, as scary to me as it was promising: I knew what kind of white noise went on in my own brain most of the time.

When you are living with pain and fear over when the next medical shoe will drop, or ruminating over your latest blood work, or worried about how you will get on a plane at six a.m. to give a two-hour talk a thousand miles away in the midst of a flare that has you so exhausted that brushing your hair feels like finishing a marathon, your state of mind is triggering a negative floating brain.

Yet, I reminded myself, this new understanding of the science of joy and well-being provides us with a powerful tool that may be able to help us retrain our mind against this damaging PIN response, if we know how to harness it.

Examples emerge everywhere in the science.

For instance, when Tibetan Buddhist monks practice compassion, or loving-kindness meditation—a meditative technique in which we send loving thoughts to those we love, those we don't know well, and even those we feel animosity toward—they generate intense gamma waves in their brains. These gamma waves are associated with higher states of mind in which we eliminate thoughts of fear, worry, pain. The most intense activity lights up the left prefrontal cortex of our brain, just behind the left side of the forehead—an area associated with joy, happiness, and positive thoughts.

Until now, we've assumed that the biggest payoff of such a brain-body practice is a better and happier state of mind in the face of life's trials. What we haven't understood is that firing up specific areas of the brain through meditation and other newly recognized approaches not only changes our thought patterns, it sets in motion a cascade effect, sending chemical molecules and messengers throughout the body that dramatically impact the action of every cell, system, and organ—and the course of our well-being and health.

In fact, the more we engage in these specific practices, the more new neural networks we create, allowing us to reset our brain. The more we practice activating states of joy and well-being, the more our brain settles on the latter as our default setting, protecting our cells and immunity, helping us to live life fully.

Likewise, fear and suffering in the face of stressful life events—including our emotions about illness—can be as damaging to the immune system as a virus or toxic chemical hit and can do similar long-term damage.

MY QUEST WAS as much professional as it was personal: I knew I was hardly alone in my hunger to rekindle a sense of joy and well-being despite the physical realities I faced. I wanted to help every woman—or man—who was wrestling with similar issues to find ways to enhance her brain's own healing responses.

I knew that 133 million other Americans—one out of two adults—suffer from at least one chronic condition: back pain, irritable bowel and digestive disorders, arthritic conditions, migraines, thyroid disease, autoimmune diseases, depression and mood disorders, cancer, Lyme disease, fibromyalgia, chronic fatigue syndrome, and chronic pain. Experts predict that these numbers, which have been rising steadily by more than 1 percent a year, will rise 37 percent by 2030.

And most of us are women:

- Women are more likely than men to suffer from migraines, and significantly more likely to suffer from lower pack pain, which is more painful in women than in men.
- Ninety percent of fibromyalgia sufferers are women.
- We are twice as likely to suffer from depression, which scientists now classify as an inflammatory disease: individuals facing depression have higher levels of inflammatory chemicals that impact the pathways of the brain as well as increase overall chronic disease risk.
- We are more likely to suffer from irritable bowel disease and arthritis.
- Women are three times more likely than men to suffer from autoimmune diseases including lupus, multiple sclerosis, type 1 diabetes, thyroiditis, rheumatoid arthritis, and inflammatory bowel disorders.
- Because breast cancer affects younger women more than most cancers, women under sixty suffer from higher rates of cancer than do men (in later years men suffer from cancer at a higher rate than women).
- We're far more likely to find ourselves facing multiple chronic conditions that elicit both more emotional distress and a greater chance of disability. Fibromyalgia *and* diabetes. Migraines *and*

slipped disks. Thyroid condition, irritable bowel syndrome, arthritis, *and* lupus. For women, diseases seem to come in pairs, or even in sets of three and four.

Recently, I sat at a conference on women's health issues, where we discussed chronic diseases with noted physicians in a variety of fields. "Walk into any of our waiting rooms and it's full of women in their thirties, forties, and fifties," said the director of one clinic. "The American woman in her prime is our prime patient; she's the walking wounded of our day." Around the table, a dozen heads nodded yes.

The walking wounded of our day.

Despite our growing numbers, we are largely invisible. Often, the illnesses women face remain unnoticed by casual observers, even those who may think they know us fairly well. According to the Census Bureau, 96 percent of us who confront a chronic health problem live with an illness that has no surface manifestation—we don't use a cane or any visible device; we don't wear a cast or bandages or appear disfigured. We seem, at first glance, to be well enough.

As a result, the daily physical, emotional, and spiritual struggles chronically ill women so often face go largely unseen and uncounted. Often, women tell me they secretly feel their illness is their personal failure. They don't talk openly to their friends or colleagues or husbands about what they're going through, and they don't know how to find one another. They're so good at hiding what they're suffering that they don't recognize each other when they pass on the street, or chat over coffee at work, or meet over the bake sale table at school.

But they do find me. In the course of my work I've met and spoken with thousands of women who live with conditions that derail their lives, draining them physically, mentally, emotionally, spiritually. I understand, when I meet these women, exactly where they are—because their feelings of loss echo my own well-masked grief.

Behind our masks, we glimpse where we've been, where we are—and our fear of what might happen to us next.

Some women share their stories with me through my Web site;

other times we talk in person. I'll be finishing a lecture and a woman will linger and begin to tell me a little bit more about her life, her story. She might tell me that she's a breast cancer survivor and is on tamoxifen, or she has fibromyalgia, or debilitating bowel problems, or chronic back pain or lupus, or recurring anxiety and depressive episodes, or excruciating migraines that nothing can cure.

Pain, fatigue, and fear, these women confide, are very distracting; they narrow our bandwidth until joy can't get in. I recall one woman putting it this way: "It's as if I've been standing outside a window and looking in for too long, watching others savor a fullness—a joy—in living I'm afraid I'll never know again."

I knew just what she meant.

We are all emotional beings living in physical bodies. All of us suffer at some point or another from the frailty of the human condition. Many women are faced with this stark reality earlier than most—in what should be the fullest years of their lives. Their hopes for a different life despite their daily symptoms, and the fear of what might come next, strike a chord, however, in all of us.

And yet one doesn't have to have faced great physical pain to benefit from the new discoveries of psychoneuroimmunology and the science of joy. Certainly many women are not in the throes of dealing with an illness or injury—but still face moments of emotional or physical suffering that block out the sense of well-being we all hunger for. Almost all of us live with our share of physical or emotional disquiet—headaches, hot flashes, rashes, that churning gut, intermittent days of sadness and low mood, or anger and loss—and all of these can keep us from living the life we imagined. These day-to-day stressors are more than enough to make it imperative that we each take the time to understand how we can better our lives through the new science of joy and find a greater sense of contentment.

HERE IS HOW this book took shape:

Compelled by my own experience, and concerned by my conversations with so many other women, as well as the Web comments I received, I set out to spend a year investigating the question of how we can search for joy despite a recurring history of pain, loss, or illness. I wanted to better understand, too, the feedback loop between how feeling better emotionally might help us feel a sense of physical relief in the face of chronic conditions. How strong was that feedback loop? Could I set my own in motion?

Of course the further I delved into this research, the more questions I had about what I was reading: how much can what we do really affect the systems of the body—especially when the physical damage of illness has already occurred? Can activating a mindset of joy and well-being help reverse or at least stop the progression of symptoms, pain, disease? Or, at a minimum, put us in a place where contentment is possible despite the physical challenges we face?

Science rarely gives us such black-and-white answers.

What we do know is that the PIN response directly impacts our immune systems and cellular activity in profound ways.

We also know from related disciplines of research that our bodies have the potential for a surprising degree of cellular transformation. Many cells in the body renew themselves on a continual basis. Our white blood cells are renewed every few days and our red blood cells turn over every few months. We create a new stomach lining every five to seven days. Our skin is renewed each month. Even half of the muscle cells in our heart are regenerated in the course of our lifetime.

But what does this really mean for those of us who suffer from physical disease? Can we really change our cellular health once disease is already set in place? Change not only our levels of inflammatory and stress markers but our blood cell counts, our pain quotient?

Could I?

As I set out on my exploration, one entirely new factor kept emerging—quite strongly. Scientists are now showing in wide-scale studies that long-ago childhood trauma and adversity play a significant role in how well our immune system functions in adulthood, impacting our lifelong health. In the process of investigating this breakthrough research, I learned things that surprised me professionally and changed me personally forever.

As I got deeper into my project, I understandably met some resistance. "I worry that this just heaps more on women's shoulders—making us responsible for one more thing," one friend who has irritable bowel and chronic migraines told me. "In addition to taking care of everyone else and taking care of our illness we have to figure out ways to feel joy no matter how bad we feel—or it's our fault if we don't get well."

I took her point very much to heart.

The science presented in this book is provocative—and powerful. So powerful it might be tempting for some to use this information in the wrong way, blaming those who are chronically ill for being sick in the first place—and for remaining ill if they can't "heal themselves."

The new science of PIN is one more tool in our healing arsenal, among many. Nowhere in this discussion is there room to imply that those of us who are chronically ill caused our own illness, or that we're at fault if, despite all the brain body methods we employ, physical suffering does not improve. In the end, no doubt, the benefits of setting out to change one's own PIN response will be different for every reader. For some women, these methods may help to bring them closer to physical healing. For others, practicing these approaches may provide emotional healing, freedom from the mental suffering that so often accompanies chronic conditions, offering them a newfound state of emotional well-being that enhances their quality of life—regardless of whether their physical condition improves. Ask any one of us who faces a chronic condition, be it physical or emotional: to intervene in the mind's orchestration of suffering—especially when anxieties flare about one's illness—is no small gift.

In the course of this yearlong exploration, I delved into the most promising of these brain-body methods, charting my experience, and providing a science-based road map of the brain-body tools, strategies, and mental energies we can all draw upon to move from suffering and pain to contentment and joy. As I charted the landscape of the interior healing capacity of our brains and its impact on our bodies, I often felt I was detailing what cartographers refer to as "sleeping beauties": those parts of the map, the landscape, that we haven't, until now, known as much about as we need to in order to better determine the course of our lives.

Throughout this book I've tried to provide a blueprint for that unknown territory, showing which approaches and tools helped me most in my efforts to feel better both emotionally and physically, so each reader might begin her own journey. What approaches made the biggest difference when I was feeling my worst? What do we know about why they work? What makes their effects so powerful? Given the busy structure of our daily lives and the limitations those of us with chronic conditions often face, how could we pull these practices into our lives in small, but life-changing ways? Exactly how did the hard work of practicing these methods pay off in terms of feeling more joy and well-being as time went by? Did they provide any palpable relief? And, did that physical relief bring, in turn, a greater sense of joy in life? What emerges throughout the course of this book is a set of tools to choose from to help you assemble your own healing toolbox.

The most important thing is that each of us sets out to discover what strategies work to maximize our brain's own healing response, and that we take time to practice these, even when we don't think we're well enough, or have time or energy enough, to try.

I want to give every reader the best possible chance to claim wholeness, leave suffering behind—and reach a new level of wellness.

In the pages you're about to read, I hope I've made that welcome outcome possible for you. It may seem an unlikely thing to wake up one day feeling joyful and alive, despite so much pain, fear, and fatigue. But with determination and dedication, I know it can happen. It happened to me.

PART I

In the Beginning

· 1 ·

The Joy Thief

I am lying on the floor at the top of the stairs, hands on my chest, knees bent. The laundry basket stuffed with clothes sits by my side.

"Mom!" my daughter Claire calls up from below. "Do you know where my lacrosse jersey is? I need it for tomorrow!" She climbs the stairs, stops at the sight of me, and leans over, her soft, brown hair tickling my brow as she peers closer. For a split second, the hanging light behind her head makes the ends seem to sparkle. "You okay, Mom?"

"Fine, sweetheart," I say. Some days getting up the steps turns my legs to taffy. Evenings are hardest. So I haul myself up by pulling along the banister, then lie down on the landing until my legs stop quivering.

"Okay, good," Claire says, looking at me harder.

"Check your drawer?" I tap her gently on the nose; it's a reflex I have whenever her face is close to mine.

Lying here for one minute more will give me the oomph to switch into manual override and keep on keeping on—critical during that witching hour when my son, daughter, husband, and I go from laughing ourselves silly at the dinner table to the homework-laundry-work-deadline-dinner-dishes frenzy. The more exhausted any one of us might be, the more likely one of us is to overreact to some small but seemingly big thing. One person's momentary brain funk can precipitate a domino effect meltdown, changing the tenor of our house from silly good humor to cranky-central.

That means when someone says they can't find their sweatshirt I hear myself groan, sigh, and say, "You're kidding me, you didn't leave it on the bus again, did you?" instead of, "Let's go back to where you had it last. . . ." The more tired I am, the less likely I am to rise to the art of grace-under-parenting.

Claire unbends her lanky body and nods, half turning to check on me one more time as she heads down the hall.

She is the first to panic if she thinks I'm not okay. Recently, we were walking the dogs when I tripped over my own feet. Sometimes I have foot drop—the sole of my foot doesn't lift up quite as far as it should and the slightest rise in the sidewalk can mean I find myself flat on my face. Because my blood doesn't clot normally, an impressive amount of blood suddenly appeared across the knees of my white cargo shorts and across my palms. I reassured her that I could easily hobble the two blocks home, but she shrieked in a panicked voice most parents only hear their children unleash in the throes of a two a.m. nightmare, *Somebody help my mommy!!!*" The lightning speed with which she hit her internal panic button—because of how often she's seen me in a medical crisis—hurt worse than any sidewalk burns.

The good and the bad news is that after what she's witnessed in eleven years as my daughter, lying at the top of the steps with my arms folded gently over my chest is nothing at all. So is falling facedown on the sidewalk, come to think of it.

I hear drawers open and close in quick succession. A second later, "Found it!"

"*Donna?* Have you seen my wallet?" My husband is calling up to me from the kitchen. "I know I left it right here on the counter, I'm sure I put it here!"

"Try the sofa?" I call. I dimly recall seeing it there next to his suit jacket, though I'm not sure if that was today or yesterday.

Footsteps. "Not there! You haven't seen it?"

I sigh. The family joke is that I possess an internal "uterine tracking device"—my husband and son rely on it to help them find everything from the ketchup in the fridge to their cell phones to their flip-flops. All day long. I would normally start searching piles on his desk, ferret through his shorts in the laundry, and find it in five minutes tops. But I can't bear the thought of getting down and up the steps again when my legs are only now starting to feel as if blood courses through their veins. Besides, I haven't given up hope he'll develop a prostate tracking device if I stop aiding and abetting. I hold out even greater hope for my son—I started his training at a much younger age.

I hear Zen still turning over stacks of papers, books. I try not to feel guilty lying here while everyone zips around the house trying to find what they've mislaid.

"Things have a way of turning up!" I say, calling down to my husband from between the banister's railings.

I stare at the overflowing laundry basket, still waiting for me where I set it down. *Keep on keeping on.* Sometimes I resort to instructing myself, as if I were talking to a small child. *You can do this. Really you can.* The familiar inward-onward charge.

Suddenly I feel all my brain-body fatigue coiling up tight inside. If my life were an economics problem it would be easy to see, black and white, the figures right on paper: daily exertion + life demands > bodily stamina.

My son clambers up the stairs two at a time and steps over me, his French book under his arm. He sets it on the floor and offers me both of his hands to draw me to my feet, though he knows that in a minute or two I will get up on my own. He is smiling—glad, I think, to be bigger than me now, stronger than me, able-bodied enough to help me out. And late in the day, I have to admit, help is nice.

"Thanks, honey," I say, as he pulls me to my feet—yanking a tad too hard. He doesn't yet realize his own newfound adolescent strength—no matter how often we tell him that the force he packs when he wrestles with his dad or bear-hugs me is five times what it was six months ago. "Watch my back!" I sputter. He tries to compensate by resettling me against the wall.

Too much. For a second I stand against the wall, eyes squeezed shut, making sure neither of my slipped disks has slipped any further.

"Sorry!" he says. His face wells up. "Sorry, Mom!!"

I lose the growl. I smile at him. He is a lovely boy. Young man. I remember him at two, planting daffodil bulbs with me in the garden, his face welling up when a bumblebee he was watching with delight turned and stung him between his eyes. When life turns from grace to pain in a flash, he takes it hard. And I have given him, I think, too much experience with that.

"All good," I say, opening my eyes.

"Can you go over my French vocab with me?" he asks.

I am glad to hear myself utter, "In ten minutes," instead of, "God help me." I head to the linen closet to stack the swim towels in a neat pile beside the bath towels.

In truth, God—or some great benevolent something—has helped me.

I know that I am a very lucky woman. I've been paralyzed twice and learned to walk again; my heart beats via a pacemaker; drugs make my thyroid work; physical therapy helps manage muscle and bladder spasms; and some of the best doctors in the world keep me going despite low blood cell counts and clotting factors and nerve damage and slipped disks and spells of recurrent fevers.

I'm still here. My children have seen it all; it's our normal. Or sort of. They know the toll illness can take on a family that loves each other. But they don't—or at least I hope they don't—know how much illness steals from me every moment, every hour.

That illness is my joy thief.

I am thinking of one Monday afternoon, a month ago.

The kids, out of school for parent-teacher conferences, are at home while I race up to Baltimore, an hour north of where we live, for meetings with their teachers (fun, because it's good news), then a meeting with my hematologist at Johns Hopkins (not all good news, so not so fun). By the time I get home I've been driving all day and fatigue reverberates through my cells. I am ready to shawl myself in my own small world. My fake-it face can't be glued on any longer.

I come in from the garage to find my son, Christian, looking somber, unusually still, surveying me closely.

"Everything okay?" he asks. "You were gone a long time."

It hits me, not for the first time, that I have spent a year of my children's lives either in the hospital or in bed—twice bedroom bound as I struggled to learn to walk again—and that several times I have gone for a "checkup" only to be admitted in the hospital and not returned for weeks.

I smile to reassure him and cover up what kind of day it has been for me, my body, at the hematology clinic.

"You're smiling—but your eyes aren't," he pushes on.

"Oh, Christian," I say, brushing back the dark brown hair on his forehead. "Am I ruining your life by being sick all the time?"

He hugs me and begins to do a slow, awkward, fifteen-year-old-adolescent boy dance with me around the kitchen. "Mom," he says, in a quiet voice, "you're giving me the best childhood on the planet. You're still here with me, aren't you?"

"You're still here with me, aren't you?" Dear, sweet, beautiful son of mine. Neither of us speaks, our untimed steps gently hitting the wooden floor. We take a turn past the stove, the humming dishwasher, the sink. In this small moment, I am not ill; I have never been ill. I am just right here, with my son. I'm not ruminating about the daunting conversation I had with my hematologist an hour ago. I'm not worried about finding that last gasp of stamina to prepare dinner or get up the stairs to bed. Every cell in my body is dancing with that incredible lightness of being that rides in with joy.

I hear lacrosse gear clatter to the floor as my husband and daughter come in the front door. As they round the corner to the kitchen, I glance up and catch a flicker of worry in my husband's expression. He's wondering whether something is wrong—perhaps my son is catching me in a fall—then our eyes meet and I see his face shift into a smile.

THESE ARE THE moments when I realize, despite all, that wholeness is possible; that even in pain one can experience moments of beauty and well-being. But it takes unusual energy and willpower to rise above the physical reality I face.

It's as if there are two different sound tracks blaring simultaneously in my mind.

The "Life Channel" and the "Pain Channel." Shutting out the thoughts that I hear on the Pain Channel—the fears—is sheer work. It's a powerful urge, to let the mind wander toward—and get stuck in—pain and worry over whether your symptoms are a little worse, even if you feel better when you don't pay them any mind. In those moments I'm struck motionless. My own life feels like it's happening at a remove—I have to work hard to reach out and grasp it.

As I am braiding Claire's hair and kissing the top of her head, I have to struggle not to register the bleak messages the Pain Channel is trying to send: the overwhelming need to lie prone; the fear that my woozy body-rush means my fever of unknown origin is now edging over one hundred degrees. I sip ginger tea for nausea and try to ignore the fact that my legs feel as alive as driftwood. I discipline my mind to focus on this glorious, delicious girl: her lit face, her animated voice. Her excitement is my anchor, my high-speed connection to the Life Channel. If I can concentrate on the smell of her newly washed hair as I weave it between my fingers, I can keep down the sound level on the Pain Channel. But it's always on, waiting for me to let down my guard.

One of my friends, a breast cancer survivor with two children close in ages to mine, says that living with the constant worry of what might happen next inside her body feels a lot like being stalked.

I get that.

I want to lose the stalker. Dial up the Life Channel 24/7. I want to walk into the kitchen and hug my son hello without his having to question every furrow of my brow, or monitor my pain. I don't want to worry that my Pain Channel has become the sound track of my family's life, too.

I want my children to grow up remembering me as the oh-how-I-adore-you mom who could. Not the mom who is always so tired, the mom who just couldn't. The mom lying at the top of the stairs.

I FINISH PUTTING the laundry away and go down to the living room to show Zen that his wallet is right there where he left it by his suit on the couch—it was hidden under his coat sleeve.

"Wow!" he says, always grateful at my ability to make missing objects reappear. I brew ginger tea for my stomach, then make my way back upstairs—slowly. I lie down in bed listening to Christian review French adjectives, then half hug, half shoo the kids into bed, before tapping out a few last work e-mails to my editors and agent and clients from my laptop propped up on pillows before me.

I read a few dozen recent studies from my journalist listserv and put several into a new desktop file I've started to create called "The Science of Joy."

These studies all emerge from a new field of research called psychoneuroimmunology, the study of how our thoughts, actions, and state of mind can trigger different immune responses. The more we experience well-being and contentment, the better our cells function. Specific approaches trigger that sensation of well-being—and better health. It's fascinating to me. And it's entirely new.

But I've hit the wall. I can feel my body and brain screaming, *Stop asking me to do more!* I shut down my computer.

Tomorrow will be another frenzied day—I meet my new internist at Hopkins because mine has recently left. I'm not looking forward to going over every nuance in my medical file. I work well with denial. Doctor appointments interfere with what I see as my primary and most successful coping strategy. Recently, I read a *New York Times* interview with the well-known doctor Julian Seifter, who suffers from diabetes and treats patients who are very ill with kidney disease: "Everyone needs the opportunity to forget their disease for a while and think of other things," he says.

I couldn't agree more. Earlier in the day I forced myself to make a list of all the diagnoses and symptoms I need to make sure my new doctor is aware of—but by the time I got to seventeen, I stopped. It was too depressing.

Light from the streetlamp outside our bedroom window is streaming in. As I draw the blinds and close the curtains before climbing into bed, I see Zen, setting the recycling out by the curb. He sees my movement in the window, and I wave down to him as he lifts his hand in his familiar gesture of half hello, half vertical I-salute-you, which always makes me laugh. He doesn't think I smile nearly enough. He spends a lot of time trying to fix that.

I hear him back inside, turning off lights downstairs. I take a sip of my ginger tea, hoping to ease my stomach pain, and look out at the quiet trees. The late May breeze brings in the soft scent of trembling leaves and turned earth, as if the rain we've been expecting all evening has already arrived.

Not so long ago I couldn't stand on my own two feet in front of this window; for months I could only see whatever slivers of life I managed to glimpse from my propped-up pillows in bed. I remember, one afternoon, after two or three months of not being able to get to the door of my room on my own, watching my neighbor's mom outside with her two-year-old grandson. She and her husband were staying for the weekend, babysitting while our neighbors were away. Her grandson, who had only recently started talking, was racing from tree to tree saying, "What this?" pointing and asking for her to name, explain. It was a glorious spring day. He didn't want to go inside. She—a young grandmother, very hip, working, on the go—was dressed for work, and she kept chasing after him in the grass in her high heels explaining, "That's an oak tree. See the oak tree? Time to go inside, Justin!" Then he'd point and race to the next beautiful thing. She would try to race after him, high heels sinking into the grass, tell him what it was, then, "Let's go inside, Justin!" This went on four or five more times before I watched her get her grandson in the door to her husband, wipe down her pumps with a paper towel, and jump in her car to race off to work.

All I could think was that I wanted that very thing back—real life. The real moment of wanting to teach a child about a tree or a bird and simultaneously feeling breathless and frustrated and rushed to get back to work, go conduct an interview, or deliver a lecture, while my heels got stuck and mucky in the damp, glossy earth. That lovely irreplaceable gorgeous mess of moment-to-moment real, ordinary life. I watched and I wept, because it was a thirst I could not quench: give me back my legs, my oh-so-ordinary life.

I thought that if I could walk on that grass again, it would be enough of a miracle.

But now I want more. I want to enjoy being right here, right now.

I know how lucky I am every time I cross the lawn, even if I'll never wear high heels again. Or each time I get up the stairs—even if I have to haul myself up by death-gripping the rail. It beats being carried up the steps in a harness slung over the back of a six-foot-three physical therapist.

I know that.

But what I've been left with is not a whole life.

That loss, day after day, isn't something I can put on a list of symptoms to discuss with any MD.

A Bold New Idea

Dr. Anastasia Rowland-Seymour, a clinician and assistant professor of internal medicine at Johns Hopkins, is accessing the hospital database on the black Dell computer mounted on a small corner desk in one of several generic ten-by-ten Hopkins exam rooms. She's reviewing my blood work and specialists' reports from the past decade. The manila patient file that sits open below with my name on it is two inches thick.

It's unlikely to faze her. Which is why my own internist, who has recently relocated to Boston, sent me her way.

I have heard Rowland-Seymour's name in medical circles for some time. Despite the fact that—at age thirty-nine—she is one of the youngest internists in the Hopkins group, word has spread that she's the doctor whom you see—or try to get to see—when Western medical care has done what it can do. She came to Hopkins after doing an integrative medicine fellowship with Dr. Andrew Weil at the University of Arizona School of Medicine. Before that, she spent most of her time working in inner-city Manhattan, getting her start in medicine working with women and children suffering from human immunodeficiency virus (HIV)—in Harlem. She walks the hard path with patients, incorporating the best that traditional medicine has to offer with alternative practices many patients have never tried or even heard of before. Although she has only been at Hopkins for a year, all second-year medical residents are already required to do an outpatient rotation in integrative medicine with Rowland-Seymour. Her practice is full, and her wait list long.

"You've been through a great deal in a relatively short period of time," she says. She looks up at me. Her brown eyes are penetrating and bright behind wire-rimmed glasses. Her shoulder-length hair, pulled back tight from her forehead into a ponytail, springs wildly free once past the confines of the elastic band that contains it.

After ten years of hospital stays I think I'm ready for any question but not the one she asks: "I'm just wondering . . . did anything happen in your childhood that could have contributed to all this?"

I'm speechless.

Nowhere in my medical record does it reveal that my father died from a medical error during routine surgery when I was twelve, or that my widowed mother seemed to disappear into her own grief.

"My dad died suddenly when I was twelve . . . he bled to death after an operation for an inflammatory bowel condition. He had the same bleeding disorder I do, and his own autoimmune struggles." I pause. "My mom was shocked and understandably quite sad and . . . everything changed." I shrug, or try to. "After that I was pretty much left to figure things out on my own."

There is so much I am leaving out: the sharp blow of loss, coming to terms with the medical error that led to his sudden death, my mother's plunge into a well of grief. An extended family imploding. Something old crosses a deeper recess of my brain, one level down.

I don't take that elevator. I blink twice.

She nods, her smile soft, as if she is not surprised by what I'm saying or that I'm leaving out everything important. It strikes me that she is not wearing the requisite doctor's white coat, but a soft, beige blouse and black slacks. "Sometimes a kind of brain-body stress—the precursor to an inflammatory response—is set in motion early on, in childhood, and we see the illness years later. What we're starting to find in the research is that traumatic events that occur in childhood can change us not just on an emotional level but on a cellular level, too."

I am staring at her, my eyes squinting, trying to follow. I expected her to ask about my sleep, my supplements. But . . . my childhood?

She tilts her head ever so slightly, as if sensing my surprise at hearing a Hopkins physician talk about mind-body from a psychobiological perspective.

"Sometimes a harmful brain-body stress cycle gets set in place during a childhood trauma," she repeats. "Or it might be triggered by present stressors, or stem from both. Whatever the catalyst, in addition to treating all the physical symptoms, we have to try to rewire the brain-body connection so that we can help to quiet that stress-induced inflammatory response, calm the immune system down, and give healing a chance to happen."

Despite being a science reporter, I find this a lot to grasp in five minutes. "Are you saying that experiencing trauma in childhood causes a stress reaction that physically changes how well our immune system functions—for life?"

"Yes," she says. "In layperson shorthand, that's exactly right."

I share with her that I've recently been reading up on how our mental state can determine the chemical signals our brain sends to our immune system, our nervous system.

"Yes," she says. "Psychoneuroimmunology. It's changing the way we look at chronic illness."

"But what you're saying is a little more novel," I go on. "You're saying that the relationship between stress and illness begins in childhood, and that what happens when we are very young might affect our immune system and our health—even decades later?" I ask.

She nods, navigating on her computer screen. "We refer to those early stresses as 'adverse childhood experiences, or ACEs,'" she explains, pivoting the monitor toward me so I can see the page she's brought up. "Researchers have been working on ACE studies for a while now. And the research tells us that childhood trauma is a strong predictor of adult illnesses." She pauses. "We're a long way from figuring out exactly what this means for patient care, though we have some ideas."

She pushes a stray, brown hair away from her face and tries to tuck it into her ponytail. It springs back. "It would be hard to imagine that your own childhood stress hasn't played a significant role in your immune dysfunction and syndromes. Your brain became wired early on to be stress reactive. Your immune system has paid the price." She pauses, her gaze certain. "It's paying it still."

"I don't see myself as someone who experienced 'childhood adversity,'" I practically sputter. Blame-the-childhood sounds like a cop-out. I'm proud of how tough and resilient I was during my childhood years. Besides, we've all had gut-it-through years as a kid. I'm not interested in blaming the problems I have now on what I couldn't control back then.

"Professional blind spot, maybe?" Rowland-Seymour muses, kindly.

"I'm trying to imagine how something happening at the age of twelve could determine my health forty years later."

"Let's put it this way," Rowland-Seymour says. She spreads her hands out in the air, giving a minuscule wave with her right fingers. "The early trauma you experienced sparked neural pathways and a pattern of hormone and inflammatory chemical cascades that have impacted you on a cellular level for decades." She pulls her right hand in, making a light fist that sits in the air in front of me. She wiggles the fingers of her left hand. "The stress you face in your daily life now from illness and any other factors adds insult to injury—sparking the same stress reactivity and inflammation cascade that was set in place early on." She pulls her left hand in and wraps it around her right hand, creating a thick double fist that looks a little like a hammer. "The stress-induced inflammatory response—and inflammatory disease—hits you twice as hard."

"You mean my stress-induced inflammatory response is stuck in the 'on' position, like a gas pedal that's always pressed to the floor?"

"That's another way of putting it." She places a palm firmly on top of the file that contains reports from every -ologist I have. "But you *can* intervene and begin to change that process now. You've tried everything modern medicine has to offer. Including a slew of alternative therapies and dietary changes. But you're not really seeing as much improvement as you'd like, are you?"

What she says is true, I admit. I've not only had a plethora of IVs and drugs put into my body, I've swallowed homeopathics and herbal supplements, and been on a half-dozen special elimination diets drinking nothing but vegetable and protein smoothies for months. I've worked with complementary health experts to detox and rid my system of everything from parasite infections to candida overgrowth to mercury toxicity. Just in case it might make a difference. And it's all helped. Here I still am. Walking. Breathing. Still alive.

But it's a getting-by life. A long way from where I might have hoped to be as a working, married, grown-up woman raising two children in what should be my most productive decades.

She drums her fingers again, her smooth brown eyes smiling. I sense she's excited—though I'm not sure why. "I know you know nearly everything there is to know about the immune system," she says. She is familiar with my last book, she says. "But what you really need to translate for people—those for whom Western medicine has done all it can—is this: all the science is pointing to the fact that your brain is your last best cure."

· 3 ·

The Cost of a Childhood Lost

When I get home, I turn on my laptop, accessing the National Library of Medicine. I easily locate the recent ACE Study Rowland-Seymour referred to and peruse the data for myself. There are dozens of recent research papers: the question of how your childhood affects you as an adult, long the domain of psychology, has, indeed, become the cutting-edge turf of neuroscientists and immunologists.

It just hasn't yet trickled down to the rest of us—even science journalists who make a living covering such things.

In a sense, that doesn't surprise me. I'm having trouble accepting the concept that our childhood can play a role in determining our adult health—and I'm well versed in the health field. No wonder the idea isn't out there for mass consumption yet.

Besides, most of the research into what is known as early life programming, or ELP, has centered on the more widely accepted concept that early physical events in childhood affect adult well-being. There is evidence, for instance, that if a mother suffers from a flu or bacterial infection during certain windows in pregnancy, her child has a higher chance of developing mental illness later in life. Low consumption of fruits and vegetables in childhood is linked to higher rates of cardiovascular disease in adulthood. If you break a bone when you are ten, it may still ache on rainy days when you are fifty. We intrinsically get the idea that *physical* events in childhood might impact our adult health.

But ACE research adds an entirely new dimension to this scientific discussion: it tells us that when something *emotional* happens to us when we are very young, it can impact our physical body at age thirty or forty or fifty or beyond, and that these emotional hits from adversity do every bit as much damage to our future health as do the physical hits we take.

As I read more about the ACE Study, here's what I learn:

The Adverse Childhood Experience Study, or ACE Study, was created to examine the precise link between childhood adversity and the likelihood of developing medical conditions as an adult. Indeed, the ACE Study, the largest scientific research investigation of its kind, has given neurobiologists a new view into how what befalls us in childhood and adolescence may linger with us forever—actively impacting the biology of our cells.

Between 1995 and 1997, health care professionals at the Kaiser Permanente Medical Care Program in San Diego, working with investigators from the Centers for Disease Control and Prevention, assessed the health status of seventeen thousand HMO (health maintenance organization) patients who came in for a complete checkup. During their physical exams, patients were surveyed about their childhood and adolescent history.

Researchers were looking to find out whether patients had grown up experiencing any of the following conditions before turning eighteen:

- Emotional or physical neglect
- Recurrent physical abuse
- Recurrent emotional abuse
- Contact sexual abuse

They also looked at whether patients had lived with any of the following individuals or conditions in their household:

- Someone who was chronically depressed, mentally ill, institu-tionalized, or suicidal
- An alcohol and/or drug abuser
- An incarcerated household member
- The mother was treated violently
- They had lived with only one or no biological parents (which would include the death of a parent)

(See the appendix on page 261 to ascertain your own ACE score.)

This was by no means a down-and-out group; this was mainstream, "successful" America: people with good educations, solid health ben-efits, and stable jobs. Participants were mostly middle or upper-middle class, and three-quarters had attended college. The average patient was fifty-seven years old.

After the interviews, each participant was assigned an "ACE score" that corresponded to the number of adverse or traumatic events he or she had experienced decades earlier, while growing up. Two-thirds, it turned out, had experienced at least one category of childhood adversity before turning eighteen years old. One in six had an ACE score of 4 or higher.

I think, for a moment, of a friend of mine, whom I'll call J. Like me, she suffers from more chronic illnesses than she can count on one hand. When J was nine, her parents split up. She spent every other weekend with her dad, who felt J wasn't nice enough to her stepmother. He threatened not to pay child support unless she straightened out her attitude. By the time J was fifteen, she barely heard from her dad. Later, there ensued bitter fights over college bills. Meanwhile, faced with the stressors of single parenting, J's mom became increasingly anxious and began to self-medicate with a scotch—or three—each night to "settle her nerves." From time to time, J would find her mom sprawled on the sofa in the morning, where she'd passed out the night before, still wearing her dental hygienist smock with her name tag on it. J once told me about how she would concentrate on the happy, lit-tle, gleaming white smiles against the green background of her mom's smock as she shook her awake.

If ever the subject of her childhood comes up in casual conversation today with someone she doesn't know well, J shrugs and says her parents divorced when she was nine. End of story.

But ACE investigators would see those years as the beginning of J's story. They would assess her as having an ACE score of 5. One point for each different type of emotional stressor she struggled against: (1) her parents' divorce, (2) her father's emotional abuse, (3) her father's neglect, (4) her mother's mental illness, and (5) her mother's substance abuse.

When researchers of the ACE Study first began assessing their seventeen thousand patients, they had no idea what they would find once they correlated the multiple categories of adverse childhood experiences, or ACEs, each individual faced, with the degree of illness he or she experienced as an adult. But when the first study results were tallied and initially published in 1998, the correlation proved so powerful researchers confessed it "stunned" them.

To FIND OUT more, I reach out to lead Kaiser Permanente researcher, Vincent Felitti, MD, to ask him about his early research findings. He tells me that "the prevalence of these childhood experiences, and their profound impact decades later, exceeded anything we had conceived."

The higher a participant's ACE score, the worse his or her adult health outcome. The correlation between having a difficult childhood and being chronically ill as an adult was profound. Researchers were at first concerned that perhaps high-trauma people like J might be more likely to engage in unhealthy coping mechanisms such as smoking and drinking, and that would account for their poorer health outcomes. But that didn't turn out to be the case. Yes, some study participants did have a higher likelihood of engaging in such self-medicating behaviors, but the evidence was clear, says Felitti, that the profound negative effect on adult health remained startlingly high even when participants did not have a history of smoking, drinking, or drug use.

For instance, those with ACE scores of 7 or higher who didn't drink or smoke, and who weren't overweight, still had a 360 percent higher risk of heart disease—the number one cause of death in the United States—than those with an ACE score of 0.

Somehow, the trauma that happened in one's childhood had a hugely damaging effect on one's later health—in a way that had nothing to do with one's own poor health habits.

Although the ACE Study did not specifically track what age groups were most likely to be adversely affected by childhood trauma, Felitti and his colleagues knew, from clinical experience, that the earlier an adverse experience occurred, the more damaging it was likely to be. This is presumably so, Felitti explains to me, because "the world is more threatening to a small child than to an older adolescent, and the earlier events occur, the more likely the brain is to be in a vulnerable stage of development." Theoretically, ACEs that occurred at the age of three were often more damaging than ACEs at the age of ten. But all ACEs mattered. And they mattered a lot.

Surprisingly, no single one of the ten categories appeared to cause more damage than the others. Although researchers anticipated that some types of trauma, such as incest, would prove more destructive, this turned out not to be the case. The one exception was that recurrent humiliation seemed to have a slightly higher statistical correlation to adult illness—which made sense, says Felitti, given that "recurrent humiliation destroys one's sense of self."

I tell Felitti a small bit about my own experiences—the death of my father, the depressed household that unsurprisingly ensued after, my recurrent hospitalizations due to autoimmune disorders in adulthood. He points me to a study he recently coauthored showing that, for each ACE score, a woman's likelihood of being ill and hospitalized with a range of autoimmune diseases increases by 20 percent. If my own ACE score is, to be conservative, a 2, that suggests that I entered adulthood with a 40 percent higher chance of being hospitalized with an autoimmune disease than someone who didn't have an ACE score.

In 2010, Felitti and his colleagues published a full review of their findings that brought a new level of attention to their work. The field of ACE research has been growing, with dozens more studies looking at correlations between ACE scores and specific diseases. Childhood adversity, it turns out, sets in place an early pattern of inflammation and cellular aging that casts a long shadow on our health. An ACE score of 6 and higher shortens a person's life span by almost twenty years. Children who have a parent die, face emotional or physical abuse, experience childhood neglect, or witness severe marital problems between parents are more likely to develop cardiovascular disease, cancer, lung disease, diabetes, headaches, and, as we've seen, autoimmune disorders like multiple sclerosis and lupus. Facing difficult circumstances in childhood increases your chances of having chronic fatigue syndrome as an adult sixfold. Kids who experience physical abuse are more likely to develop peptic ulcers in adulthood. Those who lose a parent in childhood have triple the risk of depression as adults. And children whose parents divorce are twice as likely to suffer a stroke at some point in their life.

In other words: the emotional loss we suffer when we are seven or ten or twelve or sixteen lives forever—in our cells.

I THINK, FOR a moment, of a conversation I recently had with Claire. She'd had her ears pierced for her birthday and one lobe had become infected. Although it had been bothering her for days, she didn't tell me until it was full of pus and we had to see our pediatrician. I asked Claire why she sometimes hides it when she has a scrape that needs cleaning and a dab of Neosporin, or something aches. Similar things have happened before; when she was seven she tried, with very little success, to hide a sprained ankle. The temporary subterfuge delayed diagnosis and treatment for what turned out to be a fractured growth plate. At the time, when I talked to our Hopkins-trained pediatrician, who is also my dear friend, about how much her hiding her injury worried me, she reminded me that Claire had seen me lose the use of my legs—twice—before she was six. "It's too scary for a seven-year-old to discern between one reason you can't walk and another," she said. "And the fear is there that something like that might happen to her—or to you again. Of course she's going to try and pretend any pain away."

"Mom, look at Ashlie," Claire was saying to me. I was trying to talk to her about something serious and she was telling me to watch the dog who was looking anxiously out the patio door, her ears pricked up, listening for sounds we couldn't hear.

"Claire, love," I said, trying to hide my worry and my frustration. "You need to tell me about something like your ear when it starts to bother you. The sooner we catch it the easier the fix."

"Mom, look at Ashlie! Can you see the wolf in her?" she asked.

"What do you mean?" Her question seemed so random.

"You can't see the wolf inside her, can you?" she asked. Her voice was a note higher than usual. I realized that she was trying to communicate something that really mattered to her. "You can't see the wolf in her, but it still affects what she does. Just like your being sick in the hospital a lot when we were little is still inside Christian and me. You can't see it, but it's still inside of us."

I stand there for a moment, stunned. My hand grips the counter. "I . . . can understand that," I say, groping for time, for adequate words. "Next time, when you hear your inner wolf trying to tell you what you should do, tell me, okay?" I ask, slowly.

I like to think it is a good thing that after she gives me a little done-with-that nod she asks, "Are we having that yucky grilled kale with dinner?"

THAT NIGHT, AFTER I go to sleep, I am awakened by a dream.

I am standing in the brick-floored foyer of my childhood home, painting a WELCOME HOME, DAD sign for my father. My paintbrush is thick with bright yellow paint as I spell out the words in large, childish letters, *D . . . A . . .* I can smell the rich, thick egg tempera. Slightly metallic.

I look down at my shoes. Splashes of dark red paint fall on my bright white Keds, which, in my dream, are so brand-new they almost sparkle. I am confused. I look at the yellow paint coating my brush, then down at my sneakers again. I am not painting with red. But the spots of red on my shoes expand. I look up at the ceiling, looking for the source of the red drops. But suddenly I'm not in a room at all. I'm out under the open sky. I look down again. The blood-red spreads across my white Keds.

I wake up, gasping.

My nose is bleeding, as it sometimes does at night—part of having a blood-clotting disorder. I sit up, grab the tissue box, and apply pressure to the bridge of my nose. It takes a moment for me to stop shaking. Not from my bloody nose—I am used to that—but from the dream. I tuck my hand under Zen's warm, beating chest to reassure myself that I am here, in this room, right now, and no longer twelve.

The house is quiet. I apply more pressure to my nose.

There is little chance that I'm going back to sleep.

The dream, however, is already slipping away. But something else comes in its place.

I remember.

How it went that summer day.

I *was* painting a welcome home sign for my dad. It was more than a week after his surgery. We were expecting him home in a few days' time. I couldn't wait to get things ready for him. I couldn't, I remember, bake his favorite lemon bars; I was told he wouldn't be eating normal food for a while. So I was painting a sign on pieces of construction paper I'd taped together to hang across our foyer.

Then, the news. My mother's car pulling up in front of the house, her gray-haired father driving. My grandmother following in her car. Not understanding why they'd come back from the hospital so early that morning. Why my grandparents were here at all. My mother asking my three brothers and me to join her in her room. Knowing, somehow, what terrible thing was coming before the words were born. "They couldn't help him . . . they tried. But they caught it . . . too late."

Later, over the days that followed, the rest of the news. It was a gross medical error. My father's two physicians hadn't conferred with each other. His internist had prescribed oral steroids to treat his neck pain and arthritis after a car injury. His gastrointestinal surgeon neglected to read all the file notes. He used a type of suture that was known to slowly dissolve in patients taking steroids. Post-op, my father's intestinal sutures slowly began to melt apart. After more than a week of their silently disintegrating, his bowels opened. He began to bleed profusely, developed peritonitis, went into shock, then cardiac arrest. According to the surgeon, "He could not be revived with normal measures."

Neighbors, friends, half of our town lined up to donate their blood that last awful day, but all the donated blood in the world wasn't enough to help fight hemorrhaging and an infection like that. "Normal courses of antibiotics were unsuccessful," read his death report.

So many cars coming down our oyster-shelled driveway. The phone ringing until it seemed a predatory animal. Reporters wanting to know if it was true: was the newspaper editor dead?

I'd pick up the phone, hear them asking, and put the phone back in its cradle without a sound, as if not speaking the words could reverse the truth.

JUST A FEW weeks earlier, I'd been standing with my dad at the end of our dock, his hands cupping his hips in his familiar stance as he took in the end of the day on the bay he loved. The falling light made my thin, gangly arms glow pink, like the insides of the shells we'd collect at the end of each summer along the ocean.

"Look!" he said. My father's finger charted the path of a blue heron as it took off from a driftwood tree that lay in the creek. We shielded our eyes from the hazy wheel of summer sun to watch. The heron turned on tilted wings in front of us, crossing the thin line where water meets earth, then where earth meets sky. It came so close to us we felt its blue wings beating air before it disappeared. My dad looked down at me and squeezed my shoulder. We stood there a little longer, not saying a word.

Even as it began I didn't want that moment to end.

Later, when visitors came by droves, and leaned close to talk at me, their hands bracing my shoulders, I stared out at the bay from the glass wall of our living room and pretended to hear what they had to say. Behind them, the sky seemed vacant and dull, as if a child had taken an angry eraser to the horizon.

All my life there had been a space that my father had inhabited beside me—even if he was at his newspaper and I was out riding my bike. Whether we were reading lines from Shakespeare or sitting in the cockpit of the boat as he taught me how to tack and come about, I knew he *knew* me. With him, I got to be who I was.

Suddenly that live connection went dead, the space beside me turned one-dimensional, empty, cold.

I WAS THIRTEEN when I started to have fainting spells. At twenty-eight I began having full seizures, winding up in the hospital for the first of what would be many long stays. At small intervals, my heart would stop beating. My cardiac surgeon inserted a pacemaker. Not enough oxygen, not enough life blood, pumping from my heart to my body and brain.

IS IT POSSIBLE that the research—and Rowland-Seymour—are right: the trauma of that time had played some role in the inflammation and chronic conditions I now face? I think of my ever-low white blood cell count, my damaged nerves, my eczema-plagued skin. My skin peels off. My myelin sheaths wear away. My white blood cells won't muster up to fight. Something keeps blasting away at me—from within.

Had those terrible years been brewing cellular havoc for decades?

THE NEXT MORNING, after a few hours of fitful sleep, I wake up thinking about something else Rowland-Seymour had said before I left her office: "It's never too late to intervene in the process."

After I get the kids off to school I e-mail Rowland-Seymour and tell her I'm intrigued. We agree to meet for a second time, later the next week; a visit that coincides with our need to go over my thyroid numbers.

"Are you saying that you think by employing a number of brain-body approaches we can alter the brain's state of mind and change the inflammatory patterns we set in place decades ago? And maybe even hope to change our health outcomes?" I ask her.

"We don't know all the answers yet." Her half smile plays on her face. "But we do know that trying to change the brain to a more positive state of mind will frequently lead to positive effects."

Here's what we do know:

A mindset of worry, pain, and suffering can activate the brain to send forth a brew of inflammatory chemical messengers, molecules, and hormones that cause damage throughout our body and cells. Research bears this out in myriad ways: chronic stress is linked to depression, cardiovascular disease, hastening Alzheimer's disease, and a range of illnesses. The more stressful life experiences you face—the death of a child or spouse, divorce, an assault, job loss—the more likely you are to die in the next eight years. If you're stressed or depressed, ulcers take longer to heal. A fight with your spouse means blisters take longer to mend.

Conversely, when we activate feelings of joy and well-being, we turn on a very different circuitry of healthy, positive molecular interactions—sending forth a "floating brain" of chemicals that influence and impact every cell and organ in the body. Activating a mindset of joy and well-being helps to deter the inflammatory and chemical bio-markers that promote disease. That's why individuals who regularly cite experiencing more joy and contentment have a 22 percent lower risk of heart disease.

We know that there are specific, well-researched approaches and practices that set this beneficial molecular cascade in motion, changing our PIN response. The most well-studied of these are meditation, yoga, exercise, immersion in nature, and acupuncture. In other words, we have the power to activate the protective, healing power of our brains. To send out a helpful floating brain rather than a harmful one.

"The science of joy tells us that we can do very specific things to change our PIN response, and maybe even our health," I say to Rowland-Seymour. "We don't know how much relief a patient can expect when pain, fatigue, and other symptoms cloud everything else. But I'd like to find out."

WE AGREE TO spend a year experimenting with ways to activate the healing parts of my brain. Our goal will be to engage in practices and find tools that help me to change my own PIN response and turn my floating brain from negative to positive. As I work to move my mind-set from fatigue, frustration, worry, and pain and toward contentment and joy, our hope is that my inflammatory and stress biomarkers—those associated with disease activity—will begin to quiet down. We outline a plan:

1. Dr. Rowland-Seymour will order a wide range of tests to estab-lish a baseline on my blood counts, blood biomarkers, cardio-vascular markers, cytokine, and stress hormone levels. We will ask psychologist Marla Sanzone, PhD, to help us determine the prevalence of my positive moods (joy, contentment, and well-being) and negative moods (sadness, depression, and anxiety). Her testing will provide the psychological baseline for my "joy index" as I set out on my journey.

2. We will focus on the basic approaches of meditation, yoga, and acupuncture, for three reasons. First, these modalities are available to most people no matter where they live. Second, meditation and yoga have been shown to be beneficial in terms of lowering inflammatory markers linked to virtually every disease from depression to back pain to cancer. The research on acupuncture is still emerging, with some scientists arguing that its benefits may be due in part to the placebo effect—and yet, real or placebo, people heal. Rowland-Seymour sees acupuncture transform her patients' lives. And finally, meditation and yoga can be learned without great expense through affordable community classes and supplemented with Internet downloads or DVDs. Acupuncture is usually covered by insurance.

3. I will spend a year working with experts who have trained in one of the above modalities and used them for healing in their own lives.

4. We agree that I will not swallow anything new or different. I will stay with my current supplements and anti-autoimmune diet. The supplements I take include vitamins B, C, and D, calcium, OPC-3 (oligomeric proanthocyanidin), flax, DHA (docosahexaenoic acid), and evening primrose oils. My diet emphasizes whole fruits and vegetables and excludes gluten, dairy, and additives. Should I need to receive the aid of traditional Western medicine at any point I will do so. In other words, I won't stop taking my thyroid medicine, and if I need IVIG—intravenous immunoglobulin, or infusions of other peoples' healthy antibodies—I will get it.

5. I will chronicle my journey, turning my brain and body into a laboratory as I try to change my blood biomarkers for stress, immune function, and cellular breakdown. There will be no flying off to ashrams. Everything I do will be in the context of my everyday life—a life that is complicated by my various illnesses but also by the demands of work and family. I'll keep tabs

on how much different modalities help me to feel emotional and physical relief, especially when I need them most.

At the end of the year, Sanzone will re-administer "the joy index" and Rowland-Seymour will retest all of my immune biomarkers and my blood work. She'll also conduct a full patient-doctor evaluation.

I tuck my papers under my arm and head to the front desk to make the lab appointment for my blood work.

And so begins my quest.

· 4 ·

The PIN Response

When ACE researchers first established that what occurred in our childhood could impact what later happened with our health, they were left with what scientists refer to as a scientific gap. What was the biological mechanism through which childhood trauma impacted a person's brain and body for life?

In the few years since the ACE Study was first published, researchers from the Centers for Disease Control and Prevention and Kaiser, as well as scientists from other research institutions, have continued to search out the answer to this question. And it seems to lie in the way the young brain reacts to being repeatedly thrust into a state of fight or flight.

We've all heard stories about how fight or flight can alter a person's physical state in a flash. The plot foil of a popular comic book and TV show from my own childhood, *The Incredible Hulk*, centered on just this precept: a nice-guy scientist suffers from a curse in which extreme emotional stress causes him to morph into a powerful, enormous green monster possessing superhuman strength.

We sometimes hear, in real life, the occasional news story of a person who was able to lift the mangled end of a car and single-handedly save a trapped passenger. My husband's family tells a similar tale: when Zen was two years old, an enormous three-foot-tall iron radiator weighing over four hundred pounds was being removed from his house during a renovation. Workmen left it leaning against a wall. A curious toddler, he tried to climb up on it, and it toppled on top of him. His mom pulled it up and him out. The next day it took three grown men to lift that radiator and haul it away.

Fight or flight is the reason why, in that split second, my elegant, petite mother-in-law who stands four feet eleven inches and weighs all of ninety pounds became the proverbial mother-who-would-and-could-do-the-impossible to save her child.

Fight or flight does completely alter our body—but only occasionally in ways that are quite so beneficial, or so evident to outside observers.

Usually, the effects of fight or flight are far less tangible or visible—even as potent changes are taking over our body chemistry, hormonal activity, and inflammatory processes within. Whenever we face any externally stressful event—a pink slip, a purse snatcher, the two a.m. call that someone we love has landed in the hospital—our brain instantaneously reacts. An inner alarm goes off. We go into a state of physical and emotional hyperarousal. Our heart beats faster, allowing more blood to enter our large muscles in case we need to do battle. Our muscles tense in readiness. Our pupils dilate. The hair on our body might even stand up so that we're more sensitive to vibrations in the air around us. Fat and glucose are released into the bloodstream to fuel our next move. The flow of blood to our stomach starts to shut down, leaving us with a case of "the butterflies," as oxygen moves away from our digestive tract and flows into our limbs, in case we need to strike out to protect ourselves, or take off and flee.

These responses are regulated in our body by what's known as our autonomic nervous system, or ANS. The ANS is the part of our nervous system that regulates internal functions such as our heart rate, blood pressure, and digestion. When we enter fight-or-flight mode, the part of our ANS known as our sympathetic nervous system, or SNS, revs into high gear, speeding up all systems in order to protect us. In the process, it signals our hypothalamic-pituitary-adrenal axis (HPAA) to send cascades of stress hormones through our body and get us ready for the big bad thing that's coming our way right here, right now.

Our hypothalamus, the brain's primary regulator of the endocrine system, drives the pituitary gland to prompt the adrenal glands to release the stress hormones epinephrine, also known as adrenaline, and cortisol. Our neural pathways prompt our immune cells, called macrophages, to secrete powerful inflammatory cytokines such as IL-6 and IL-2 that whip up the body's immune response. This floating brain of neurochemicals charges through the body at split-second speed.

The good news, for my husband, is that the day the radiator fell on him, his mom's ANS, SNS, and HPAA (the whole alphabet!) kicked off in perfect working order, allowing her to lift four hundred pounds and help her toddler son to crawl out unscathed. Her stress response served a protective function in the face of an emergency—a threat to her son's life.

The problem is that in our modern life we often feel as if life-or-death danger threatens us around every corner. Yet most of the "danger" we face is far from potentially fatal. It's more often emotional: lost keys, traffic gridlock, a cutting remark that steams us. But the stress response still kicks in, as if lost keys or a spouse's criticism might actually spell the death of us. Yet fight or flight is hardly an appropriate response to these more pedestrian situations.

As a result, we've become a little like cats living in the midst of a neighborhood of imaginary barking—even snarling—dogs. It doesn't matter if the dog is large or small. An altercation with a coworker can cause the stress response to kick in. Or getting an unexpected bill in the mail. Or seeing a car swerve in front of us. So can just thinking about any of these things happening, or ruminating over them after they've occurred.

It is enough for us just to feel that a threat looms near. In his book, *Full Catastrophe Living,* Jon Kabat-Zinn, PhD, the pioneering architect of what's known as the mindfulness-based stress reduction program, one of the most widely studied and successful programs ever developed to help reduce patient stress reactivity, cautions that "the mere *thought* that you have a fatal disease can be the cause of considerable stress and could become disabling, even though it may not be true."

Over time, most of us have come to accept life in a state of chronic hyperarousal. For those facing a long-term medical problem, the pain, worry, and fear that accompany any illness are added triggers, one more fear-making situation sending the SNS into overdrive.

Kabat-Zinn points out that nature intended for us, after entering a state of fight or flight, to release all that stress from our bodies by physically exerting ourselves until we reach a state of exhaustion. After we fight or run, our heart rate returns to normal, our breath, blood pressure, and blood flow readjust. Our muscles relax. Oxygen returns to our digestive tract. We begin the process of recovering and restoring balance in our body.

But we rarely react in physical ways to the mundane stresses of our modern world. We don't take off racing down the street or hit a punching bag after we find out we didn't get the job we wanted or that our boyfriend cheated on us or that the lab test came back with less than stellar news. We internalize the stress we feel, holding it tight in our muscles and bodies. We suppress our feelings. We pretend we are fine. We say we are fine.

As Kabat-Zinn says, "We put the arousal in the only place we can think of, deep inside us." We carry on, business as usual. We never get to experience the physical release and recovery phase. Instead, we stay incredibly tensed up as we encounter one dangerous-feeling threat after another. It becomes our way of life.

But it doesn't have to be that way.

The autonomic nervous system also regulates the part of our nervous system known as the parasympathetic nervous system, or PNS. The PNS is the yin to the SNS's yang. It is often referred to as the "rest-and-digest" system. It's meant to be our day-in, day-out baseline—the calm state of homeostasis and balance from which we experience occasional stress spikes of hyperarousal. When our PNS rules, our body, brain, and mind enter a resting state that allows us to experience a sense of relaxation, tranquility, and contentment. We experience a feeling that all is well with the world that frees us up for the *aha* moment, creativity, love. The PNS is the Life Channel. Literally: take away our PNS and we can't breathe and our heart can't beat. We die.

To keep all this straight it helps me to think of the SNS as the stress-now system, and the PNS as the purr-now system. Corny, but there it is.

Unfortunately, for most of us, the sympathetic (stress-now) nervous system has, instead, become our baseline. Day after day, we overreact; the SNS fires away; and the negative floating brain runs rampant with inflammatory chemicals and cytokines through our brain, organs, and cells. When our negative PIN response stays high for extended periods, it wreaks havoc on the body. This leads, over time, to the long-term physiological damage and chronic inflammatory health problems so many of us suffer from, including high blood pressure, stroke, diabetes, depression, autoimmune disease, asthma, bowel issues, and heart disease.

BUT SCIENTISTS ARE coming to realize something more perturbing. When, like my friend J, or perhaps, like me, we are repeatedly thrust into a state of hyperarousal when we are still young and our brain is developing, the physical and emotional sensations of fight or flight do more than send forth a toxic floating brain cocktail that surges into the bloodstream and body.

At McGill University, neurobiologist Michael Meaney recently found that this chronically elevated state of fight or flight causes deep biophysical changes in the young, developing brain. This occurs through a process known as epigenetics: biological changes that affect the expression of our genes—in this case, the genes that govern our stress hormone receptors in the brain.

Here's how epigenetics works. Every cell in the body has the full set of chromosomes and contains all of our DNA. But the reason why one cell, during embryonic development, becomes a skin cell versus a bone cell or eye cell is because most of the genes that could be expressed are turned off. They get switched off by an epigenetic process called gene methylation in which small chemical markers, or methyl groups, adhere to specific genes, silencing them. This gene silencing is permanent, which is why we don't grow eyes in the back of our head. But scientists are beginning to realize that the brain is an epigenetically "privileged" place. This process of DNA methylation can occur much more easily within the brain, allowing the brain to respond to experiences that might be good or bad, and change with those experiences over time.

Meaney has found that when the young, developing brain experiences ACEs, these small chemical markers, or methyl groups, adhere to specific genes that oversee the production of stress hormone receptors in the brain. These chemical markers disable these genes, preventing the brain from successfully regulating its response to stress long into the future. The chemical markers that should govern stress hormone production profoundly disregulate the brain's ability to moderate stress—and they impact us for life.

This methylation process tips the brain into a state of constant hyperarousal. Stuck on autopilot, inflammatory hormones and chemicals keep coursing through the body, like a leaky faucet left on, building up corrosive effects that, as the years tick by, have far-reaching and lifelong mental and physical consequences.

By the time children with a high ACE score reach adulthood, their stress hormone and fight-or-flight responses have been stuck in the "on" position for decades. They may grow up to be hypervigilant, seeing threats where none exist, overreacting to confrontation, showing increased aggression, or responding to small altercations as if they mean life or death. Or they might react in the opposite way: under-recognizing dangerous or unhealthy situations, and entering relationships and situations that are chaotic and harmful because they seem familiar and safe.

The good news, says Meaney, is that his rat studies indicate that these methylation patterns can be ameliorated by healthy, nurturing parenting. This means, hypothetically speaking, if J's mom had been nurturing and present enough to support J through her hurts and frustrations in the face of her dad's emotional abuse and neglect, J's brain might not have been at high risk for this methylation process and epigenetic changes. But because no one was there for J, chances are quite good that her brain experienced this methylation shift. Her negative floating brain got stuck on autopilot. Inflammatory hormones and chemicals kept coursing through her body, year after year, building up toxic effects that, over time, became damaging to her on a cellular level.

Researchers at Harvard have done similar groundbreaking work, showing how early childhood stresses rewire the circuitry of our brain, changing our epigenetics, and altering gene expression. They also found something else I find quite staggering. ACEs cause profound physical changes to the area of the brain that processes our emotions and our memories, known as the hippocampus. According to Harvard researchers, experiencing physical or sexual abuse, physical or emotional neglect, significant separations or losses, verbal abuse, or parental discord during childhood results in having a smaller hippocampus— about 6 percent smaller than that found in adults who didn't experience these forms of childhood adversity. It seems that a group of cells in the immature hippocampus releases a hormone when faced with excessive stress. Exposing the developing hippocampus to large amounts of this hormone reduces the actual size as well as the function of the emotional processing center of the brain. This damage to the hippocampus and our ability to process emotion, which in turn impacts how we react to and manage stress for life, may also help explain why early adversity often leads to a multitude of later health problems.

Research in this area has come so far in such a short time that, as we've seen earlier, scientists can now speak directly to links between adverse childhood experiences and dozens of specific diseases— including all three of the syndromes my friend J currently suffers from: rheumatoid arthritis, an autoimmune disease; migraines; and irritable bowel syndrome.

For instance, compared to people with no ACEs, someone with just two ACEs in childhood is at a 100 percent increased risk of being hospitalized with a rheumatic autoimmune disease decades down the road. I wonder what J's chances would have been of developing rheumatoid arthritis if she had had zero ACEs instead of five.

In 2011, the American Headache Society devoted a good portion of its annual scientific conference to observations linking adverse childhood experiences to the likelihood of having migraines in adulthood. One of the physicians presenting at the conference stated that clinicians were "finding an unusually high prevalence of childhood abuse in migraine patients." Again, the ACE data bore this out in a clear dose-response relationship: as an individual's number of ACEs increases, his or her risk of suffering from migraines increases proportionately. And—perhaps unsurprisingly, given the way the PIN response causes oxygen to be diverted away from the intestinal tract— there is a direct correlation between childhood trauma and neglect and the likelihood of developing irritable bowel syndrome.

In a sense, by the time my friend J was fifteen years old, she barely stood a chance of being a fifty-two-year-old woman in good health.

It is much easier for me to think in terms of the research and, especially, how the research affects others.

It is far harder, however, to think of how it might apply to myself.

I GET IT, intellectually, that the links among childhood adversity, the negative floating brain, and adult illness are increasingly spelled out in the pages of scientific journals. I know that Rowland-Seymour suspects that the sudden loss of my father and the traumatic years that followed may have triggered a chronic pattern of stress reactivity in the pathways of my young brain. And that, in turn, has played a role in my body's cellular breakdown from my neurological to gastrointestinal to cardiology systems, not to mention my largest organ, my skin.

But that doesn't mean I want to turn the microscope there. And I don't want to blame my childhood for any aspect of my life now. That seems a slippery slope away from self-responsibility I don't want to skid down.

Still, if I want to help counter the adversity my own kids face having a mom whose energy flag is at half-staff, and if I want to heal in my own right, then I probably have to look at my own past and consider patterns of mind I may have set in place early in life that are causing me to be overly stress reactive in my adult life. And I probably have to take responsibility for my role in how that happened and in how I might reverse any negative patterns that were previously set in motion.

I'VE ALWAYS THOUGHT of the events of my childhood in terms of *how life turned against us*. My dad's sudden and inexplicable death, my mom's own terrible sadness. My family falling apart. I've never thought about that time in terms of *how my brain might have turned against me*.

If I have to turn my gaze back to those years, then I want to do so with equanimity. Without blame.

Those six years. Twelve to eighteen.

No one predicted my dad's death; no one expected it. Some extended family members wanted to sue the hospital; others, including my mom, thought it unseemly, something nice people didn't do.

It was the 1970s; no one spoke directly about what had happened, much less about grief. "Talking it out" wasn't yet in the cultural lexicon and "How do you feel?" was not a question people in a nice Episcopal family like mine asked unless we were feverish. We were reassured that our terrible sadness would end in about six weeks—that was the appropriate time frame—after which we would feel significant relief.

That Rx didn't work for me. Six weeks later I was living in what felt like a postapocalyptic world. A very, very quiet postapocalyptic world.

My mother cried in her room; I cried in mine. That's how things were done back then. My brothers fell in love and began hanging out at their girlfriends' homes and rarely at our own, and who could blame them? A family of six diminished into five separate satellites. I rarely saw my older brothers anymore. They had two distractions and escapes I didn't: love and wheels.

Now, decades later, married to Zen, whose family is Japanese, I have learned that the Japanese culture doesn't have a specific word for grief. Neither did our family culture.

We each found our own coping mechanism. My brothers played music, spent time with girls. Mine, in the interminable quiet and feeling of aloneness that was left to me, was to slowly imagine my father back to me.

I find myself embarrassed to admit it now, but there it is.

My dad, I told myself, would never have abandoned me without saying good-bye. How could he?

In nights of magical thinking I talked to him, getting through long, sleepless hours by imagining him there by my side. I felt him; I certainly thought I felt him, in the same way you suddenly know, without turning around, that someone has entered the room. It was different from his really *being* there. Still, if I were very still I felt I could sense his soft, familiar comfort. *I'm here. It's okay. Things will be all right.* When I felt it I knew. That feeling couldn't be wrong, could it?

One evening as my grandmother passed by my door, she heard me talking aloud to the empty air. It shook her. She sat down on the side of my bed and asked me if I really understood that my dad wasn't ever coming back again.

Of course I knew, I told her, too ashamed to share my secret conviction.

Meanwhile, when I was around other people, living people, words wouldn't float up out of my throat. So began my silent year. A few of my teachers had their eyes on me, maybe because the sudden death of my young father—editor of the local newspaper—had been big news. My seventh-grade social studies teacher had us perform our oral reports one day, and when I choked and couldn't get further than the first sentence, he told me to try again tomorrow, rather than deflate my grade. But he didn't make me get up in front of the class again.

Another afternoon my English teacher, Mrs. Lindow, gestured, "Come with me." She ushered me upstairs to the third floor to the teacher's library and told me, "Whenever you want to, you can come in here and get any book you want." She pressed into my hand my own small, silver key. Her chin-length, dark brown hair framed her small, earnest, heart-shaped face in perfect symmetry, curving neatly down like two parentheses.

She stood there for a moment, and I knew there was something more she wanted to say. "I admired your father, Donna," she said. "He was a good man. He did good things for this town." I gave her the same mute nod I gave everyone that year. I knew he had meant something to more people than just me. I knew from the fact that the church had been standing room only at his funeral, the crowd overflowing out the front doors onto the lawn. I knew from the people who came up to me on the street to tell me about the time he'd helped to bring their son home from the Vietnam War, or made a few calls to help their husband get the job that kept them from losing their house, or been so willing to go up against petty mafia types in the pages of the newspaper that he was once shot at through his windshield (they missed on purpose, people said—though we did have to stay home from school for a few days as a cautionary measure). Or that the night Martin Luther King Jr. was shot he walked the most dangerous streets of the city until dawn with our local black leader, trying to calm fears and keep our streets from breaking into riot. I knew that he had had a role in our community that was bigger than his infinitesimal role as my dad.

But that was the only role I cared anything about. I missed perching on the ottoman next to his chair at the end of the evening, telling him about the latest drama with my friends at school—two friends warring with each other as girls do and trying to get me to side with one or the other. "Why don't you go to school tomorrow and get each of them to help you do something really nice for the other," he'd say, "and see what happens?"

Or, if we were sailing and the night sky was at its peak, "If you were sitting on a planet way up high, looking down at this tiny boat in this big bay on this huge planet, your problems wouldn't seem so big, would they?"

I have wondered, looking back, if he was thinking then of his own growing worries and pains.

It never occurred to me to wonder, in the years he was alive, if I was protected, out of harm's way.

In my postapocalyptic world I'd curl up with my cats. I'd had my tonsils out at the age of five when the surgeon discovered with a shock in the operating room that I had the same rare bleeding disorder as my father. I'd bled so severely that I'd spent days and nights in the hospital. I recall vomiting blood. My dad, allergic to cats, promised that if I got better I could finally have the kitten I'd been asking for, as long as it stayed out of his room.

After Smokey came Tigger, a fat and happy tabby. Then Dilly, a willowy calico always at my heels, waiting at the end of the driveway when my bus pulled up. When I did my homework, Dilly would sit on my shoulder, pouncing down to bat at my pencil as it arced across the page. When Dilly had kittens in my closet, I kept a black and white with a bright pink nose and named him Captain.

When magical thinking and my cats weren't enough, Mrs. Lindow's small, silver key provided escape through the novels of Edith Wharton, Henry James, James Joyce. Being handed that key was one of the great kindnesses of my childhood. A year or so later, another teacher stepped in—my art teacher. I began to spend lunch hours painting in her art studio. A few years later, it would be she who took me on my college tour, who told me I could move on with my life, though we never discussed what it was I wanted to move on from.

She seemed to know, without knowing, that something was wrong with me. The sadness that emanated from me like dim oil light. Maybe she suspected that at home really difficult things were happening.

And they were. Instead of helping, family members had swooped in, more interested in father's business interests than in the wife and children he'd left behind. We had, suddenly, very little income for a widow and four children. The boats were sold. My mother wasn't herself—who would be, husband gone overnight? She had no one to talk to or lean on. She woke up one day widowed with four teenagers to take care of. Friends disappeared.

We kids all got jobs. I worked in a crafts store on weekends; at the public library every day after school, shelving books in the children's section; and as a bus girl bussing tables at an Italian restaurant, where we dressed up in Colonial pinafores and servant's mobcaps.

While the grown-ups were busy being angry with each other, there were no grown-ups to lean on. My dad had been the glue that had held to keep old family grievances at bay so the family didn't explode. Without him the explosion just kept on going.

Everyone made me angry. I worried about everything. I worried about my mother, who seemed so bitter and angry and sad. Was she ever going to be okay?

Looking back, I don't know how she had the courage to keep on keeping on. How she kept our household going. But she did. She took classes at a local college. She got a job as a bookkeeper. She tried not to let the free fall her life had taken bring her to her knees. How brave she was.

She paid the bills. There was food in the cupboards.

But things were hard. She had no one to lean on. No one at all.

Not long after my dad died I came home from school and Dilly and Captain, who usually met me at the bus stop, weren't there. Usually, when my feet hit the driveway my cats would weave in and out of my legs, their tails conferring small comforting taps on my shins as we walked the gravel drive home. I called for them for hours, walking into the woods and swamp and even down to the water's brink, where they would never go. They didn't come. I knew something was wrong when my brother came down to the edge of the woods and put his arm around my shoulders. He told me that my mother had all four cats put to sleep that morning because one of them had been peeing in the living room. It had been the last straw for her. The one more thing she just couldn't take.

No discussion.

Were those years enough to change my brain for life? Would a researcher say my score for adverse childhood adversity, or ACE, was high?

I've never thought of my childhood as traumatic. But now I am not so sure. It seems likely that, for me, small methyl groups adhered to my genes in such a way that it altered their expression, preventing my brain from successfully regulating my stress hormones for life.

A LITTLE PERTURBED by all that I've learned—and concerned that it might be too late to change the brain that I now have—I reach out to neuroscientist Margaret McCarthy, PhD, professor and chair of the Department of Pharmacology at the University of Maryland School of Medicine. McCarthy conducts research into how epigenetics impacts nuances of behavior and mental health. The good news, she reminds me, is that the brain is an epigenetically privileged place not just in terms of creating negative changes, but positive ones as well. "Our brains are malleable," she reassures me. "Scientists are now of the mind that DNA methylation can come and go. And it may be that the reason why approaches such as meditation and mindfulness have such power is that they undo bad epigenetics or even induce new, good epigenetics."

I like that. Our current behavior *can* rewrite our epigenetic future. We can do something about the impact our ACEs have had on us, even decades after the fact, and begin to amend our biological glitches, no matter what caused them. We can start wherever we are.

The more I learn, the less willing I am to accept that my life now should feel like my life when I was twelve. The more determined I am to change.

· 5 ·

Baseline

The Hopkins lab has seventeen vials of my blood. So much that after drawing the first nine vials the woman in the lab had me leave for an hour, drink a gallon of water, and then come back and sit with a heating pad on my arm until she could find a vein that was still good when she tapped it. I've also had my saliva swabbed for three days straight so that we can assess my cortisol levels. The results, when Rowland-Seymour calls me one night to go over them, are a little more disturbing than I might have liked.

One aside here: I have found, over the years, that when a physician calls you after five o'clock at night it is generally never sensational news.

I know that I often have less than pretty blood work. I know some of it is troubling. My hematologist has looked at my blood cells under a high-powered microscope, which reveals that my red blood cells are larger than normal. In addition, some of my white blood cells, known as neutrophils, contain discolored dohle bodies, which are very rare and indicate some type of chronic inflammation. He even had my three older brothers send him blood samples to see whether mine represented some kind of genetic mutation within our family. It didn't. It's just me.

And I have known for some time that starting about fifteen years ago—the furthest back that we have records for it—my white blood cell count, or WBC, has been quite low. The average WBC ranges between five and ten thousand. Mine has ranged from one thousand (when I was paralyzed) to a little over three thousand. This is not great because white blood cells fight infection. That means that when I have a cold, it doesn't last a week. It lasts a month.

"Right now your white blood cell count is 2,500," Rowland-Seymour says. "Your absolute number of lymphocytes, or the total white blood cells counted, should be between 120 and 300. Yours is 20."

Meanwhile my red blood cells are being pumped out of my bone marrow too fast, and are a little too big, which tells her that my bone marrow is working extra hard to make them.

"Your mononuclear cell count is high," she says. "Normal is between two and eleven. Yours is over fifteen." She pauses. "This tells us that you're responding to a chronic disorder of some sort."

My iron count is a little low as well—and I'm not storing iron well. My iron levels should be between fifty and seventy and mine are twenty. My ferritin level—which measures how well my red blood cells are storing iron—should be between ten and three hundred. Mine is four.

My complement factor is also quite low. This matters a lot. Complement factors—called C3 and C4—"complement" the work of antibodies in destroying foreign invaders. "They act like a kind of glue, allowing our fighter white blood cells to stick to abnormal proteins so they can annihilate them," Rowland-Seymour explains. "When you're fighting some kind of foreign invader nonstop, your complement levels go down—because all the complement factor, or glue, is being used up as your white blood cells adhere to the bad abnormal invader cells and try to eliminate them."

I think about this for a minute. "So, my army is running out of the regular supplies it needs to do its job on a continual basis?"

"Well, in a sense, that's right."

My salivary cortisol levels are high. Very high. Salivary cortisol measures how much stress a person is having in the here and now. Normal range is between 0.04 and 0.56. My levels, taken on two different days, are 0.73 and 0.95. Off the charts. "Salivary cortisol levels in this range tell us that you are currently feeling an acute level of stress right here, right now," she says.

Another stress marker, IL-6, which measures our inflammatory cytokines—the chemicals that whip up the body into an autoimmune or inflammatory response—is not as elevated as we might have expected. Mine is 0.44, moderately high. But another similar cytokine level, IL-2—also used to measure cytokine activity and inflammatory processes—tells a different story. Thirty-eight and up is elevated. Mine is thirty-eight. So my IL-2 cytokines are circulating heavily. They tell us that I'm experiencing chronic, long-term stress.

A negative floating brain of neurochemicals is coursing through my body on a regular basis.

My antinuclear antibody (ANA) count, which looks at antibodies that are turning against the body itself and harming one's own tissues, is slightly positive. It's not high, but any ANA count at all can point to an autoimmune process. Mine is forty and what they call "slightly speckled." But I don't need to worry that it speaks to lupus or mixed connective tissue disease . . . my numbers are below that threshold.

What's going on with me is something else entirely.

"And, so," I say, a little dumbfounded, "what do you think all this points to?"

She clears her throat, taking a minute before she speaks. "What I believe these peculiarities mean is that there is some ongoing, chronic autoimmune process taking place that is causing your bone marrow to produce cells less efficiently than it otherwise would," Rowland-Seymour says. "But what that is . . . we have no idea."

I feel a little flattened at her pronouncement. I'm setting out on this journey to heal my brain and hopefully help my body—but right now I feel as if the mountain is way too steep and jagged for me to climb. How can I pump up my bone marrow in the face of whatever mysterious chronic thing it's fighting by using modalities as simple as meditation, yoga, acupuncture, and nature walks? Which leads to my next question.

"We have no idea what my bone marrow is fighting?"

She must suspect how I'm feeling. "No," she says. "What I want you to remember is that despite all this you're doing . . . okay."

"I don't know if 'okay' is the right word." I try to laugh.

She laughs with me. It's reassuring. "Point taken," she says. "Let me see you next week and we'll run a full physical exam in my office, and get a read that way too."

NOT SURPRISINGLY, TEN days later when I see her, our list of medical diagnoses is fairly stark:

Vasovagal syncope, a fainting and seizing disorder, treated with a pacemaker.

Small-fiber sensory neuropathy, or an autoimmune disease of the small sensory fibers in the body that help us to feel heat and cold and to manage and hold objects in our hands. (There is no treatment, one just has to live with that dead feeling in one's hands and feet, and with dropping things left, right, and central.)

Pancytopenia, which refers to those low white and red blood cell counts.

Von Willebrand disease. Lack of sufficient clotting factor in the blood. It is why some women used to die in childbirth, and it's why at any given time I have small bruises on my body, and why minor surgery for me is never a minor thing. Happily, synthetic hormones work to clot my blood—but they cause other problems, so my hematologist tries to avoid them whenever we can.

Thyroiditis. Solved, more or less, by taking thyroid hormone pills each morning. Though anyone with a thyroid disorder knows I'm making light of this.

Guillain-Barré syndrome, twice, which has left me with nerve damage in my extremities, muscle damage, and spasms that are treated with physical therapy. GBS is why a few days ago a teacup flew out of my hands and landed on my wireless computer keyboard, so that the only letter the keyboard now types is *P*. It's why our rescue pup, Ashlie, the corgi-Chihuahua (we think) watches me cook and chop—hoping for scraps—from just outside the kitchen doorway. She knows knives and other small items like garlic presses sail from my hands with no warning and these mysterious flying objects can nail her, scaring her so much she quivers for twenty minutes afterward. It is why I fall over my own feet and hold on to people when I get up from a chair or have to step over something on the ground or walk up and down bleachers at lacrosse games or track meets.

To test my balance, Rowland-Seymour asks me to walk across her exam room with one foot in front of the other in a straight line, as if doing a drunk driving test. I can't do it. Not even for two steps. She catches me in free fall before I crash, careering sideways, into the exam table.

She also has me walk on my toes in her office, which is hard for me, though I do my best.

The next day I feel the exercise keenly, when both of my calf muscles seize up. If I exert a select set of muscles strenuously it can cause them to turn rock hard and sore. Whenever I complain about this to my neurologist, he reminds me that I don't have all of the normal nerve connections left in the muscles of my body. When most people use their muscles, they use one set of nerve connections and, when those are spent, they draw on another. But my body has only a limited set of nerve connections to draw upon. When I use them up, that's that. If I keep on trying to use them, my muscles lock down, quiver—they let me know they are done. There is no second or third set of nerve connections for my muscles to tap into to power up.

There are still so many other things on the symptom list.

Muscle weakness after short exertion—some days just getting up a steep incline in a parking lot makes me feel so spent I can't walk for one or two minutes. Many would call this chronic fatigue—the feeling, sometimes after simply getting up off the sofa, that every sinew, muscle, blood cell, synapse, and nerve has been usurped by some other force, my own life force stolen away. But for me it may be a matter of nerve damage. Either way I often feel throughout the day that I would feel better lying down.

I also have a long history of bladder spasms and pelvic floor muscle spasms; this requires more physical therapy, exercises, and stretches.

And then there is my back. A few years ago our one-hundred-pound golden retriever pulled me down the front steps in a serpentine twist and I slipped my L3, L4, and L5 disks and injured my sacrum, pelvis, and sacroiliac (SI) joint. I've had weekly physical therapy ever since. At last, something normal, Zen joked, trying to make me see the humor in finally having a midlife ailment that others would recognize by name.

Then there are the gastrointestinal issues. After I had GBS the second time, I ended up in the hospital in a gut-related crisis. The gut is full of nerve endings—that's why we get "butterflies" when we're nervous or feel fight or flight—and mine were compromised. Things didn't motor through my gastrointestinal tract as they should, which led to intestinal infections and a year of antibiotics. Now, eating a special whole-foods diet, I wrestle with more minor episodes of what is classically known as irritable bowel syndrome, or IBS. With, in my case, a little nerve damage complicating things. Some days it can be debilitating.

I also have chronic tendonitis in both wrists and hands. Basically my tendons are chronically inflamed. Wearing wrist braces to type helps.

We talk about my history of fevers of unknown origin—for a year or so my temperature would spike up to one hundred degrees for no good reason.

And then there are the skin rashes. A seemingly small thing on the list but one of the things that drives me the craziest. The burning, itching sensation is so constant, irritating, and disruptive it wakes me up through the night. I have eczema on my face all the time. Both eyelids are scaly and red. My chin sometimes swells up like a puffer fish. The skin between my nose and mouth scales off every few days in white flakes. If you walked by me in a crowd you might think I have some rare skin disease. It makes me so self-conscious that sometimes I keep my dark glasses on inside so at least my red, crusty eyelids can't be seen.

Anyone who has ever had eczema knows what I mean. Sometimes I have it in the crooks of my arms, on my neck, or my hands. It waxes and wanes but never really goes away—especially on my face. My dermatologist once said, "Remember, this is a minor problem compared to everything else you've been through." But it doesn't feel minor. *Scratch, scratch, scratch.* And the topical immunomodulator creams used to control the autoimmune process behind eczema cause other immune side effects that my dermatologist doesn't like, so they are out for me, though I'm told I can use them in advance of special occasions, for one week only, then stop. I have long thought that if all of my autoimmune eczema cleared up, without using creams, it would mean that I was becoming healthy inside. That something enormous and seismic had changed within.

Insomnia. If you've ever had it you know what I mean.

Headaches. They come and go.

I fill out an inflammation index with over two hundred questions to help get a sense of what symptoms of inflammation bother me most in the day to day. My numbers come back glaringly high in the following areas: numbness, fatigue, skin rashes, gut issues. My total inflammation score is ninety-six. One hundred is considered severe. Zero to ten is ideal.

I never before looked at my physical conditions altogether like this. I've tried not to be so . . . comprehensive.

As diagnoses have stacked up, I've adapted to each new condition, accommodated myself to living with a little more numbness, a little more scratching, a degree more of fatigue, and more back pain and bowel issues, accepting the newest ailment or pain quotient into my repertoire, subliminally factoring it into my awareness of what I have to get up and work around each day. After a while, my memory of what I felt like before that newest physical glitch grows foggy.

• • •

IT'S AN ALP to climb, to try to combat all this with state of mind and see if we can get to the other side.

Meanwhile, Rowland-Seymour has it all in my file now—which is suddenly much thicker. Blood work, symptoms, inflammation scale. We have quite enough to use as a point of comparison to reassess where I am in a year versus where I am now.

WE CHAT FOR a moment about our goals in terms of the practices we will choose for my yearlong experiment. We reiterate our three primary objectives. We will focus on approaches that are (1) supported by current scientific literature and her clinical experience, (2) available to people no matter where they live and without great expense, and (3) gentle enough that most people, even those with limitations, can engage in them.

"Where would you like to start?" Rowland-Seymour asks.

"Meditation," I say. "The literature on how meditation and mindfulness maximize the healing responses of the brain has been so compelling." I'm hopeful that they can help me to reverse the negative stress-reactive processes in my brain that have long been set in place. I find myself deeply drawn to the idea of trying to sit and quiet my mind, I explain. I'm hungry to find out what it might be like to even momentarily silence the Pain Channel at will.

"Let's begin with the inside—the brain—and work our way out to the body," Rowland-Seymour suggests.

"Yes," I agree. As we talk, our plan emerges. I will spend the first half of my year—the fall and winter—attempting to alter my PIN response by trying to change my interior mental activity, and the manner in which I respond to life around me, through meditation. My efforts will center on a technique known as mindful breathing—a meditation approach in which we move our attention away from our spinning thoughts, using the breath as an anchor to help calm the mind. I'll also explore loving-kindness meditation, or compassion meditation.

After I establish a solid practice in mindful breathing and loving-kindness meditation, I'll spend the second half of my year—the spring and summer—exploring yoga, laughter yoga, exercise in general, and acupuncture, and the role these might play in redirecting our floating brain and PIN response. At the end of my year, I'll evaluate what tools are working best for me and why.

I decide not to confess to Rowland-Seymour how scared I am that none of this will work on me.

But I think of my children, of how their "normal" is having a mom who lies on the floor at odd times. Of what my illness—the joy thief—has already robbed from them, when their idea of a good childhood is simply that I'm still alive.

I don't want my Pain Channel to become the childhood pain that keeps them from the Life Channel— now, or twenty years from today. There has to be a better way.

PART II

Meditation:
Coming to the Quiet

Mind-Full

The first time I meet Trish Magyari I am late. Her office is located in an old, historic manor home in Baltimore, which has been renovated to house dozens of practitioners' offices. Despite her careful directions I have trouble finding the large white mansion and locating the right entrance. When I get to the top of the stairs, I head in the wrong direction, which means I end up outside a nutritionist's office. By the time I double back and arrive at Trish's office, I'm five minutes tardy and my legs are wobbly.

"You found us," she says. "I'm so glad. It can be tricky to find." She extends her hand, her voice warm and welcoming. Her chestnut brown hair is clipped short in a pixie cut. Seeing that Magyari is in her socks, I slip off my sandals before entering her office.

She gestures to two chairs that sit in the center of the room, facing each other in the early September light that cascades in through her office window. A set of brass-colored, sand dollar–sized cymbals lies on her chair. She picks them up and holds them in her palms, the leather cord that connects them dangling slightly, her fingers half covering the ornate markings.

Magyari sees me looking at the cymbals. "These are tingsha bells," she explains. "I use them at the beginning and end of meditation to deepen our sense of being present and here." She pauses. "Before we talk, I'd like to start with a few minutes of mindful breathing."

I nod, feeling a little schoolgirlish as I sit in my wooden chair, not sure what to do next with my hands, my eyes, my feet.

She closes her eyes and knocks the gold bells together gently. "Allow yourself to follow the sound of the bell until the end."

I close my eyes. But I am not really listening to the bell's ring. I am, suddenly, thinking of the automatic car door lock on my car. It broke this morning. I rushed out the front door into a sudden summer downpour, my computer bag, purse, jacket, and water bottle in hand, only to find the key's unlocking mechanism didn't work. I had to put everything on the wet ground. Once I turned the key in the lock and got in the car, clutching everything, I spilled half of my water bottle in my lap. My pants are still musty and damp. *Idiot*, my mind intercedes with what has almost come to seem a pet name I call myself.

I find myself reliving the hour-long drive here, combating beltway traffic, frantically finding the right staircase, mustering my legs to move faster . . .

Magyari prompts me again. "Follow the sound of the bell until it ends, allowing the sound of the bell to call you fresh into this moment. Feel yourself right here, right now, your hips and legs settling into the coolness of this chair, on this Tuesday morning." I urge myself to listen. I think of the tuning fork my doctor puts to my ear when I'm having my hearing tested. I have an artificial eardrum in my left ear, so I have my hearing tested fairly often.

I realize I've tuned out the bell again.

By the third stroke I get it. At least a little. I listen to the ringing disappear. And as I do, it comes, a tiny sense that my body really is here, in this chair, right now, with nothing to claim my attention but the bell's clear, simple chime. It's a lovelier sound to hold on to than the chatter in my brain.

She suggests I put a hand on my belly and feel it fill slowly with air. "Bring your focus to your breath; experience your breath as it fills up your abdomen." She takes in a deep breath and I join her, tuning in to the feel of my belly rising and falling with each inhalation and exhalation.

"If your mind wanders, just come back to the rise and fall of the breath, giving it all the attention you might give to watching a newborn child."

Her image helps. A lot. I feel my shoulders fall. A little.

"Let's practice a mindful sigh, letting go of everything that may have preceded being here, all the doing that came before this moment." She takes in a deep breath and heaves out a sigh so ripe with frustration, fatigue, and fed-up-with-the-world-ness it surprises me; her exterior exudes such calm. Hearing her helps me to let go with my own the-world-is-too-much-with-me sigh. Or groan. Or hybrid.

"This is an exercise known as three mindful sighs," she says, as we continue to breathe. "Research shows it helps us to let go of our thinking and physically reverse our stress response, calming down the sympathetic nervous system."

It does feel releasing.

By the third sigh some tether is being snipped to the overwhelmed feeling I carry with me . . . all the time.

My cell phone rings. It's in my purse, at my feet. My eyes fly open.

"Even as we hear sounds that may distract us, we can stay with the breath," she says, softly. There is no tone of admonishment except for the lashing I am giving myself in my own mind. "We can acknowledge the sound and let it go."

But I know Claire is home alone for a brief stretch, and she has an anaphylactic peanut allergy. I know she would never eat anything without checking with me first . . .

"I'm sorry," I say. I feel terrible, but I'll feel worse if I don't answer. "My twelve-year-old is home alone."

She opens her eyes and smiles gently as if to say, *Go ahead. It's really all right.*

"Home," the incoming call message says. I answer to hear a loud, high-pitched, frantic voice in my ear. "MOM! . . ."

"Claire? Claire—are you okay?"

"WHERE ARE MY HORSE BOOTS?"

She helps out at a barn on weekends. Her boots are new; she saved up Christmas and birthday money to buy them. She loves those boots and I can't imagine that Claire, a born finder-and-keeper, can't find her boots. But I can't solve this one from an hour away.

"Okay, go back to where you last had them."

"I had them on Saturday," she says, a whine helicoptering through her voice. Then a pause. "Ohhh no, Mom," she says. "I put them in the back of your car. I forgot Dad was taking me to the barn today!" Her voice gets higher. "MOM, THEY'RE IN YOUR CAR!"

"I'm in Baltimore, sweetheart." I pause, letting the words sink in. "Remember? I'm an hour away. You'll have to use your old boots. They'll be fine."

"AUGHH!" This exhalation of righteous hysteria, worry, and indignation is one only a twelve-year-old girl can make.

"They'll be fine. I have to go now. I love you."

"Mom!"

"You'll be fine."

"Mom."

"Bye, honey. Love you."

I HARDLY KNOW what to say to Trish Magyari.

"I'm so sorry."

"Can you give a word to what you are feeling?" she asks.

I think about it for a second. I think of being late. My damp pants. My phone ringing, interrupting. The boots in my car. My distressed daughter hoping I can fix it. My hoping I can fix it all. Disorganized me. A familiar sense of self-flagellation pulses through me. "Embarrassed?"

"What other descriptive words come to mind?"

"I'm an idiot." I smile.

"Self-judging?"

"Yes." I think about that. "Yes, lots of self-judgment."

"Try naming what you're feeling and letting it be, and then coming back to the breath." She closes her eyes again and I close mine.

I try it. I name the feeling "self-judging." I feel my breath rise again in my abdomen. It feels good, concentrating on the breath, the small movement of my lungs expanding, the air passing through the back of my throat. It is relieving, somehow, to focus on the simple words that name my feelings, rather than on my sweaty, red-cheeked sense of embarrassment. Something infinitesimal changes. Like putting a period at the end of a sentence that says, "Moving on."

It feels good. I pick up the breath.

"When your mind wanders, simply name the habit of mind and come back to the breath."

We do this for three or four more minutes, during which time I ward off perhaps a dozen "How could I have?" thoughts with "self-judging!" as if the words serve as a mental flyswatter. When Magyari rings the bells again, I am not focusing on the breath and my mind is nothing close to quiet, but I am also not feeling so much like an idiot. And that small change impresses me.

As does the graceful, concise way she has taken me from harried and self-lashing to calm and . . . right here.

The tingsha bells ring again, as a sign that our brief meditation has come to a close.

We open our eyes and smile at each other—and I realize I am smiling my first genuine smile of the day.

EARLIER IN THE week, I learned about what brought Magyari, who serves on the faculty at the Johns Hopkins Bloomberg School of Public Health, to focus her research and practice on patients like me who face chronic health challenges. In addition to teaching mindfulness-based stress reduction, or MBSR, courses, leading a local meditation practice group, and working with mindfulness in her clinical counseling practice, Magyari has been part of research teams at both Hopkins and the University of Maryland on how meditation and mindfulness help to lessen emotional and physical symptoms in the chronically ill, including female patient groups suffering from post-traumatic stress syndrome, and men and women with rheumatoid arthritis.

"Was there anything in particular that put you on this path?" I asked her when we spoke by phone a few days ago.

"I didn't have a choice," she told me. "Twenty years ago I found myself facing a level of exhaustion and pain that interfered with every aspect of my life." At the time Magyari was young, single, and working "impossible hours meeting back-to-back deadlines." Suddenly she developed the symptoms of both chronic fatigue syndrome and fibromyalgia. "I went from working full-time to part-time. Then I had to stop working entirely."

Her tone is somber as she describes those days. "I spent a lot of time managing my symptoms—and an equal amount of time managing my fear that I'd never be well again. I felt as if I were scratching my way out of a deep hole to get back to my life."

Her disability was so crushing that nothing else registered: she was overwhelmed by her pain. "The skill I honed that helped me climb my way out was mindfulness," she explains. Her words seem carefully thought out. "It was the tool in my toolbox that made recovery possible. It allowed me to occupy another, less reactive mental space. It's not a cure-all. There are still difficult days of fatigue. But my emotional and physical challenges have a different start point and a different end point. My distress doesn't rise to the same level."

In 1999, Magyari reentered the workforce full-time, working in genetic counseling at the National Institutes of Health (NIH). She also underwent formal training to become an MBSR teacher. She soon found an opportunity to weave mindfulness and her genetic counseling expertise together. One group she worked with at NIH was composed of patients who suffer from a genetic disease known as Ehlers-Danlos syndrome, or EDS. Patients with EDS have a defect in the connective tissue that gives support to their skin, muscles, and ligaments. They have fragile skin and unstable joints—the result of faulty collagen, the protein that acts as a kind of binding agent in our body, adding strength and elasticity to skin and muscles. Patients with EDS often have debilitating musculoskeletal pain, terrible bruising, and joints that easily dislocate.

As coordinator of a study that followed patients longitudinally through their life cycle to better understand EDS, Magyari began to ask herself if MBSR could help these patients who "were suffering and in a lot of pain" experience less physical and emotional heartache. She arranged for a clinical pilot study to look at what might happen when patients with EDS were taught to practice mindfulness.

As in many studies of meditation, patients learned and practiced mindfulness through an MBSR curriculum developed by Jon Kabat-Zinn, PhD, director of the Center for Mindfulness in Medicine, Health Care, and Society at the University of Massachusetts Medical Center. In the course, which has been adapted for secular audiences from its Buddhist roots, students learn a variety of mindfulness practices to reduce stress through quieting the churning mind and calming the nervous system. These include mindful breathing, loving-kindness meditation, and noting our own moment-to-moment experiences, especially our habits of mind. In the process of learning these and other mindfulness techniques, one learns to separate oneself from one's thoughts so that normal stressors no longer cause the same physical and emotional stress reactions. The sympathetic nervous system, or what I like to call the stress-now system, quiets down. The parasympathetic nervous system, or what I like to call the purr-now system, begins to hum, bringing us back to a calm and balanced state both physically and emotionally.

Kabat-Zinn has found that participants who undergo the eight-week MBSR training period in his clinic experience a significant reduction in the average level of pain they feel. In one study, 72 percent of MBSR patients with chronic pain conditions achieved at least a 33 percent reduction in their pain rating index, and 61 percent of the patients with pain achieved at least a 50 percent reduction.

The results of Magyari's study of EDS patients were similarly striking. "We saw an impressive outcome in which patients experienced less depression, anxiety, and pain." But the thing that moved Magyari most, she explains, was that "the MBSR class gave people I'd followed for years who had felt hampered by this condition the momentum to move forward toward their life goals. To start living again." Several life transformations were profound. Particularly clear in Magyari's memory were "several young women who wanted to be mothers but who weren't moving in that direction. After the course they became pregnant and had healthy babies." Other patients moved to homes that better suited them, or changed jobs. "MBSR not only helped them to heal physically but to heal emotionally—to reclaim their lives. To witness the power MBSR had in the lives of other people, people who were facing so much pain, was very powerful and beautiful to see."

One 2007 study Magyari coauthored found that patients with rheumatoid arthritis who learn and practice MBSR over a six-month period experience a 35 percent reduction in the psychological distress, anxiety, and fear that so often go hand in hand with the illness. Several patients were able to lower pain levels as well. Just as important, she says, "Those who took part in the study gained a stronger ability to cope with the physical pain that might not go away."

She underscores that this healing takes on different forms for different people: "Not everyone who is facing a chronic illness will recover on a physical level, but even recovering on an emotional level can dramatically change your life."

Other recent studies she's facilitated have used mindfulness training as an intervention for women who have survived childhood sexual trauma and who suffer from posttraumatic stress disorder as a result. "When you suffer from PTSD it's hard to live in the present; the mind gravitates to memories of the past and fears of the future."

These were women whom we might assume to have very high childhood adversity experience scores, or ACEs. No doubt many of them as children experienced the neurobiological process of gene methylation that we've examined in earlier chapters: in the face of trauma, small chemical markers attach to the specific genes that orchestrate stress hormone production, altering the ability of those genes to moderate stress hormone production for the future. The PIN response becomes chronically elevated, causing the negative floating brain of neurochemicals to course through the body unchecked.

So these women were a particularly challenging group. Yet after eight weeks the average participant experienced a 65 percent decrease in the symptoms of PTSD, including depression and anxiety. Their brains were plastic enough to still win out over chronic emotional distress.

"Many women who took this class began healing after decades of pain," Magyari recalls in a deeply caring, almost maternal-sounding voice. "The program was incredibly transformative for them." Some women called it "a new start" in life. "The women worked hard and were rewarded with a greater ability to relax and enjoy each moment. They began to have more energy, self-acceptance, and confidence."

As I SIT across from Magyari now, I wonder if she will ever be able to say anything remotely like that about me. It seems best to confess my self-doubts to her right up front. "I think I may have a meditation disability," I tell her. My determination to start this process with utter honesty overcomes my chagrin. "My mind's speedometer runs at about 150 miles per hour. I'd even say I have a dangerous mind," I continue. "I churn out worried and negative thoughts all day long. I'm not sure if mindfulness-based stress reduction can retrain a brain like mine in a body like this—and reconfigure all that faulty wiring in between."

She laughs gently with what I am coming to see as her trademark kindness. Magyari reassures me that she has a perspective on my fears—especially in the face of managing a set of physical conditions that can be both daunting and distracting. "I think for right now we should start by working on your ability to be friendly to yourself," she suggests. "Maybe by congratulating yourself for taking this time to come here to nurture yourself today."

She pauses and waits.

I must look a little blank.

She smiles her minuscule smile and pauses before suggesting that we meet again privately as coach and client prior to my starting her eight-week mindfulness-based stress reduction course. She'd like to see me soften my resistance to being compassionate to myself and learn to be more mindful of my negative habits of mind. She explains: while having difficulty in being friendly to oneself is common among those of us who have grown up in Western culture, where achievement is more important than nurturing the self, her sense is that my resistance is particularly strong. Addressing that will put me in a better position to take her mindfulness program and reap the most benefit.

We agree to meet in two weeks for a one-on-one session. In the meantime, she suggests I read a book called *Radical Acceptance*, by meditation expert and psychologist Tara Brach. She also asks me to think back to the ways in which I may have coped with any big stressors I met in my own childhood, and how I learned to relate to myself in the face of them.

I joke with her, as I am leaving, that I hope I can "remediate myself." Before the words are fully out of my mouth I realize, with a lumbering turn in my gut, that I've just given her more proof that I clearly have the habit of mind of being unfriendly-to-self. That realization makes me feel even less friendly to me.

· 7 ·

Meditating: The Sweet Spot

I am hardly unique in my joyless distraction. Most of us spend about half our time thinking about something other than what we're doing at any given moment, and most of this ruminating makes us feel pretty miserable. We know this because two Harvard psychologists recently took it upon themselves to figure out how much time we all—unhealthy or well—spend thinking about something other than what we're doing, and how being ruled by a ruminating mind makes us feel. They used a special iPhone Web app called Track Your Happiness to catalogue a staggering amount of human distractedness: they gathered 250,000 data points on people's thoughts, feelings, and actions as they went about their daily business.

It turns out that our mental lives are pervaded, to a remarkable degree, by "the nonpresent." These researchers go so far as to say that mind wandering is an excellent predictor of people's happiness quotient; how often your mind leaves the present to dwell on things that aren't actually happening in your here-and-now environment is a better predictor of your happiness than the activity in which you're engaged. They sum it up thus: "A human mind is a wandering mind, and a wandering mind is an unhappy mind."

Other researchers tell us that although 70 percent of our day is relatively good, 28 percent of it neutral, and only about 2 percent of what happens to us actually bad, we think about that negative 2 percent almost all the time; it's what we ruminate over as we shower, drive, and fall asleep. It reminds me of that old saying that we wear 2 percent of our wardrobe 90 percent of the time. We button ourselves up in our misery cloak a lot.

I think of something Pema Chödrön, the American Buddhist nun, teaches. She quotes Alice in *Through the Looking Glass*: "If you drink much from a bottle marked 'poison' it is almost certain to disagree with you, sooner or later."

It may take time. But if we busy our mind reliving the more upsetting moments of our day and react to so much of what happens to us as if it's life or death, if our body sips on that toxic cocktail that's being sent forth from the toxic floating brain hour after hour, it is almost certain to disagree with us, sooner or later.

On the other hand, I know that when I am fully immersed in who and what is really in front of me—feeling the wind rustle my hair, watching my children race into the ocean waves—my symptoms fade. My whole body smiles. My cells seem to smile. I can do more. I am more.

This doesn't mean my physical reality is different. I can recall years ago, playing the *Game of Life* with my children. I was recently home from the hospital and in bed. I couldn't walk and didn't know if I ever would again. At one moment I turned my head to sip from the glass of water on my nightstand. When I looked back I saw the kids had stockpiled my "car" with a dozen extra "babies" to take with me on my trip through life. I laughed out loud so hard—more at the conspiratorial exchange of glee on their sibling faces than anything—that game pieces rolled off the bedcovers onto the floor. Six-year-old Claire, howling, rolled off the bed onto the floor, too, and her brother followed for good, dramatic measure, with a thump and a guffaw.

I remember being surprised, in the moments afterward, at how that full-body ripple of joy momentarily released my body. My legs were still cold and blue and numb, but I felt, in that small moment, that they were also alive, tingling. I felt that I would be okay, that with a great deal of good luck and strenuous physical therapy, my legs might begin to wake up and I would get out of that bed. The possibility of healing felt real, no longer so remote.

Feeling better mentally opens the door to the possibility of everything, including physical relief. And feeling even the hope of physical relief brings me closer to a mindset of emotional and mental well-being. Which, in turn, allows for more physical healing. One can't be separated from the other. I suspect that for most of us who have been worn down by chronic symptoms and conditions for years this is, to some degree, the case.

Enter meditation and mindfulness, the sweet spot that can help us to activate that feedback loop at will, in any situation of our choosing. We focus on our breath and quiet our mind, which in turn lowers our PIN response, creating more mental space for joy, hope, and contentedness. Which sends forth our positive floating brain, bringing us a greater sense of physical well-being. Which leads to experiencing more contentment and joy in our lives. Which loops us back to that better, healthier state of mind.

The problem for me is that this feedback loop has been, to a large degree, rusting away for decades.

If I want to better connect the dots between how my emotional state impacts my sense of physical well-being, I need to better understand that link. If I am to create a toolbox that evaluates which approaches make me feel more joy and contentment, and whether feeling better mentally helps me physically, I want to understand more of the science that speaks to that deeper interplay in my cells.

Most of the broad-strokes research being done on activating the robust healing responses in the brain through meditation and mindfulness training, and how it helps to correct our biochemical reactivity and reverse the negative floating brain, has been done primarily on willing college students at university and research centers around the country.

University researchers evoke the stress response by asking study subjects to solve impromptu mental arithmetic problems in front of a disapproving panel of judges, or to give a public talk right on the spot. Often, study subjects undergo an "anger recall interview," a tape-recorded interview in which an experimenter pushes subjects to recall in detail a painful time when "they were really angry at something or someone" until the subject reexperiences his or her angry emotions as if the infuriating situation were happening all over again, in real time.

After subjecting participants to these and other stress triggers that pump up the sympathetic nervous system, researchers look at the effects on their bodies by evaluating their heart rate and taking blood samples to assess their stress hormones, immune function, and cytokine level.

They get a pretty good picture of their PIN response.

Participants then start a course in which they learn mindfulness-based meditation techniques: focusing on the breath and using mindfulness to help bring them back to the breath. Six or eight weeks later, they undergo the same battery of testing a second time to see whether what they've learned has helped them to deescalate their PIN response and bring down their inflammatory markers.

These studies are the reason why we know that meditation and mindfulness techniques bring down the PIN response, helping to reverse anxiety, depression, fatigue, and a host of chronic diseases from depression to heart disease.

Now researchers are examining how shifting our state of mind creates these positive physical changes in our cells.

Much of this newer research focuses on a particular measure of cellular health, called telomeres, or sequences of deoxyribonucleic acid (DNA) that sit at the very tip of each cell's chromosomes. Telomeres act as protective caps at the ends of our DNA, much the way the bound tip at the end of a shoelace protects it from fraying. Telomeres shorten as we age. Eventually they become so short that the cell no longer functions. The length of our telomeres is thought to be a rough measure of the age and vitality of our cells, which in turn may be linked to living a longer, healthier life. For example, people with shorter telomeres are at greater risk of depression, diabetes, obesity, osteoarthritis, osteoporosis, and heart disease. Not surprisingly, they die younger.

However, telomere length doesn't decline at the same rate for everyone. We could be thirty but have, deep within, the cells of a fifty-year-old. Or we could be sixty and have the cells of someone a decade younger. This might be because telomere length is somewhat malleable over the course of our lifetime, depending on our early experiences, lifestyle choices, and attitudes. For example, adults with a history of childhood adversity have shorter telomeres than those without an ACE history, suggesting, say researchers, that what happens to us before age eighteen has "profound effects on biology" and our most basic "cellular mechanisms"—leading to pronounced and accelerated aging.

This doesn't surprise me. Having awakened one day at age twelve to a world in which my father was dead and our family blown apart, I think it makes perfect sense that when we are very young and experience such loss, our bodies might suddenly become far older than we are.

Nor does it surprise me when I learn that being female is yet another risk factor for having shorter telomeres. We know that emotional stress takes a greater toll on women's cellular health than it does on men's. When we face acute stress, or when our stress response becomes chronic, our adrenal glands produce a more ferocious negative floating brain and PIN response than do men's, pumping a more damaging chemical cocktail through our bodies. This is related to women's higher rates of depression, cardiovascular disease, and other inflammatory and autoimmune disorders.

Fortunately, we may have some amount of control over our telomere length. Telomere length is related to lifestyle choices, such as exercise and diet. But researchers are coming to understand that our attitudes and perceptions may also affect telomere length: one study comparing the DNA of mothers caring for disabled children strikes me as particularly provocative. Researchers found that the longer a woman had taken care of a disabled or autistic child, the shorter her telomeres were—even after they corrected for a woman's age. Some mothers were years older than their chronological age.

But here's what really stands out: the more a mother *perceives* herself to be under heavy stress, the shorter her telomeres are. Surprisingly, some moms of disabled or autistic children who face a great deal of objective, real day-to-day challenges—but who don't perceive their life situations as highly stressful—do not show the same significantly shortened telomeres as other moms in similar or even less demanding situations. In other words, it wasn't how emotionally and physically demanding a mom's caregiving situation was that determined her cellular well-being; it was how she felt and thought about the situation she faced.

To get a better understanding of this mind-body relationship, researchers have been looking at how changes in our psychological attitudes and perceptions influence our cellular vitality during meditation practice. To find out more, I get in touch with Clifford Saron, PhD, an associate research scientist at the Center for Mind and Brain at the University of California, Davis, who has been leading a wide-scale investigation into meditation and its effect on brain, mind, and body, known as the Shamatha Project. Saron and I chat early one morning—six a.m. his time in California. He and his colleague Tonya Jacobs, PhD, and a large team of collaborating scientists have been evaluating the types of psychological shifts that regular meditators undergo in their thought patterns as they move away from negative and ruminating thought patterns, and whether this is related to biological mechanisms that have the potential to affect cellular health. They looked at the effects of meditation on an enzyme called telomerase, which has the ability to lengthen our telomeres. They found that over the course of a long meditation retreat, meditators began to feel more emotionally stable, were less likely to experience negative emotions, and began to perceive themselves as having more control over their lives, regardless of their circumstances. And they began to feel an increased sense of purpose. At the end of the three-month meditation retreat, these psychological changes were related to greater levels of telomerase. In other words, the more a meditator's psychological state improved, the greater his or her level of telomerase activity. Although scientists are not sure whether short-term changes in telomerase activity can directly predict telomere length over a longer term, these effects do show that our thoughts have the ability to affect the workings in our cells.

"When we pay attention and start watching the quality of our experience," Saron tells me—how upset we get when someone speaks to us in a disrespectful way, how much we let reactive thoughts dictate our feelings and sense of self—"we begin to notice gaps in our thoughts." Gaps between what's going on in our mind and what's actually happening right in front of us. "We can then deconstruct our experiences, deconstruct our reactive responses, and reconstruct our experience through the new view we gain by paying attention," he explains. "We dismantle the habitual assumptions we make between cause and effect. As we change our habits of mind we change our view from within. We change the entire way we see our world."

"The good news," Saron emphasizes, "is that we are not our thoughts."

IF WE ARE not our thoughts, then we can change our thoughts. And if we can change our thoughts, then perhaps we can change our cells.

It may even be that meditation triggers what researchers refer to as "pathways of restoration and enhancement," not only boosting the parasympathetic nervous system, which down-throttles the fight-or-flight response, but actually stimulating the production of growth hormones linked to the preservation and maintenance of each cell.

In simplest terms: the way in which we mentally perceive the stress we face and how we rehearse it in our mind may have a more profound affect on the health of our cells than the amount of stress we're actually under. And the more we move our state of mind away from negative, spinning thoughts about our life situation by focusing on our breath and mindfully bringing ourselves back to the quiet again and again, the longer our telomeres may become—and the greater our longevity.

This is pretty inspiring.

I like the idea that my brain talks to my DNA. And that if I search out joy and well-being, the healing responses of my brain will begin to stimulate the preservation of my cells in ways that extend my cellular expiration date. And mine. The more I perceive that my life is really okay, despite quirky blood cells or wobbly legs, the more my cells restore and rejuvenate.

MEANWHILE, OTHER RESEARCHERS in the field of psychoneuro-immunology are measuring how meditation strengthens the very white matter of our brains.

"White matter" refers to the brain's myelin—the insulation that wraps like a protective coating around our nerves. Myelin makes it possible for neurons to send messages from one part of the brain to the other—like a superhighway communication system, connecting the major "gray matter" regions. Gray matter, made up of neurons, includes areas of the brain involved in muscle control, sensory perception such as seeing and hearing, memory, emotions, and speech. White matter carries nerve impulses between these gray matter regions and helps our nervous system to send signals throughout our body. When the brain's myelin, or white matter, is compromised, messages become garbled.

White matter is damaged in conditions such as multiple sclerosis, vascular disease, and AIDS. Aging, arteriosclerosis, and even recent viral infections can contribute to white matter atrophy. Chronic migraines also damage white matter—especially in the female brain.

In my own life, myelin damage from GBS is thought to play a role in my leg weakness, numbness, and fatigue, and in tripping over my own two feet.

So I am particularly interested in work showing how meditation and mindfulness alter white matter. Just six hours of meditation training and eleven hours of practice have been shown to strengthen the white matter tracks in brain regions that help to govern our emotional reactivity.

This research on white matter sheds light on why so many studies indicate that meditation improves concentration and other self-regulatory skills. Students who take a ten-minute lesson in mindfulness meditation stay less stressed during high-stakes math exams, scoring on average five points higher than other students. Individuals trained in meditation perform significantly better on all standardized tests of attention. Adolescent boys who take four forty-minute classes and practice with a CD eight or more minutes a day not only improve concentration skills and math scores but experience a greater feeling of well-being, lowering their levels of stress and anxiety. And it doesn't just improve concentration in the young. Brain imaging shows that meditation also protects against the cognitive declines that occur with aging. In one recent study, while nonmeditators showed typical age-related declines during attention tests, as well as losses in their brain's gray matter, regular meditators showed no decline in the area of the brain associated with attention and concentration.

There is one other piece of literature that stands out to me, having to do with the gray matter area of the brain that processes memory and emotion: the hippocampus. Remember earlier findings that those with ACEs also have smaller hippocampuses due to the early impact of stress on the volume of the brain? Well, meditation and mindfulness lead to increases in the volume of gray matter in the hippocampus—the area of the brain that sustained so much damage in childhood. Participation in mindfulness-based stress reduction programs is associated with "changes in gray matter concentration in brain regions involved in learning and memory processes, emotion regulation, self-referential processing, and perspective taking."

As we change the view from within, we literally increase the areas of the brain that have to do with helping us to have a broader perspective on life.

This new research on telomerase and white and gray matter in the brain sheds new light on why medical conditions ease and concentration increases with mindfulness meditation. They tell us that as we learn to change our view from within, and become better able to modulate our emotional response to everyday stresses, we not only decrease the inflammatory response, we change the brain. Our white matter, which protects the nerves in our brains, will strengthen. So will our gray matter. Our telomeres will lengthen.

We can save our cells, and save ourselves.

Let's say you tend to feel anxious and keyed up whenever you talk to a particularly difficult family member. Every time you hear her voice you feel like she has a hold on your internal organs and is squeezing tight. Or maybe it's that colleague who knows you need to leave by 5:30 to pick up your daughter but who habitually tosses you last-minute projects you have to sign off on at 5:25. Or when you first take note of a flare-up symptom—an inflamed joint or a wave of flu-like fatigue—which tells you that you're not going to get much done today. Again.

Meditation and mindfulness training help you to become aware of what's happening with more objectivity so that you can step off that downward thought track. Skip the *I hate her! Him! No! Not this!* Engage in less agitating and ruminating; feel less heart pounding and stomach twisting. Loosen the noose of those added-on poisoned resentments, worries, judging and blaming, worst-case scenario fantasizing, and all the stuff that generally makes you feel like you can't breathe.

It doesn't mean the stressors go away. It doesn't mean that you don't take action and do what needs to be done. It just means you handle the situation with more awareness and creativity. With practice, you slowly become more aware of the patterns of your habits of mind, recognizing that the intense feelings you're having will eventually go away. And in the process of learning how to step away from those add-on thoughts and simply focus on your breath again, your parasympathetic nervous system kicks in, your PIN response goes down, you stop sending inflammatory chemicals throughout your body, your telomeres may lengthen—and, over time, the white matter tracks in your brain grow more resilient, thicker, and stronger. You may even reverse negative epigenetic changes that have taken place in your brain as the result of past adversity or trauma, and create good epigenetic changes that help to re-regulate your stress reactivity. You stop blocking the healing power of that happier, more joyful floating brain.

The research on mindfulness and meditation gives us hope that we can intervene, stop our mental chatter from taking over our lives, engage in what's really happening right now, and feel contentment, even joy. It tells us that so much of our unhappiness and angst—regrets about the past, disappointment about the present, fearful fantasizing about the future—is constructed by the mind. Composed by us.

· 8 ·

A Little Self-Love Here

When I get in the car and head up the highway to meet with Magyari for a second time, it's one of those days: my get-up-and-go has got up and fled. It's hard to find the oomph, physically, to drive the drive—though I've been looking forward to this all week. Luckily, anticipation douses a modicum of my exhaustion.

That isn't always the case. Many days my fatigue causes me to cancel things, or to not say yes to events in the first place—which is very different from saying no. No means no I won't or I can't. Because I prefer to think I can, I often say, "I'm not sure yet," because I don't know how I'll feel when it's time to head out the door.

Rowland-Seymour has cautioned me that when your bone marrow works twice as hard as other people's to produce half as many blood cells, and your central nervous system functions on only partial connectivity, you are going to take the hit somewhere. On a bad day, like today, the combo effect feels like my body is trying to drive sixty miles an hour in first gear.

I HAVE AN hour ahead of me on the highway to do a mental review of the two homework assignments Trish Magyari gave me when last we met.

I've read *Radical Acceptance*, by Tara Brach, PhD. Brach, a therapist and leader in the mindfulness movement, writes about how those of us in Western culture often have a particularly difficult time sending kindness to ourselves because we carry a deep sense of unworthiness within. As most of us move through our relationships, our work, even the most rote moments of our day, we're unconsciously managing a chronic sense of self-dislike.

At first, I'm not sure I buy the overall concept that we all brim with self-disaffection. In fact, I don't.

If I were to ask myself, "Do I like myself?" my answer would be—perhaps too glibly—"Of course I do." I'm very loving with my family, and I know how to say I'm sorry. I tend to be very helpful to those in need; in fact, one of my brothers tells me that being "too nice" is my "fatal flaw." Hmmm. I'm not sure, then, if that counts as something I like about myself, or something I don't like. I think of other strengths: I have made it through some hard years, hard loss, and I've come through. I think of a grade school essay Christian once wrote in which he said, among other things, "My mom is the most determined person I know. She's more determined than Frodo."

Of course he has no idea how many times I've given up, been bested by the joy thief. Slipped into the car in the garage in the middle of the night in my pj's, made certain the windows were rolled up tight, and sobbed over the steering wheel until the sight of my red, snotty face in the rearview mirror startled me. Then walked back upstairs and climbed into bed to wake up the next day and try to make gutting it out look effortless again.

True, faking it isn't the same as liking yourself. *Maybe if you liked yourself you'd be less of a fake.*

But surely it's something.

Still, as I read further, I'm surprised to find that I relate to so much of what Brach has to say. She posits that most of us in Western culture don't receive the kind of unconditional love that we long for, or experience feeling seen or heard for who we are inside. This creates a sense of loss that begins at a very young age.

She shares a story of a small girl who is tugging and tugging on her daddy's pant leg when he comes in the door from work, impatient to show him that she's written her name for the very first time. He's talking on his cell phone, pacing the floor. She's pulling at the knee of his trousers, trying to show him the work of which she's so proud. Finally, he looks down at her and says with exasperation, "What are you *doing* down there?"

"Daddy, I *live* down here," she says.

Most of us grow up feeling, in some measure, that no one is taking note of what we have to offer up to the world. From the time we are very small, we try to compensate by competing and striving hard to prove that we're worthy enough to be noticed, to belong. Cute or sweet. Smart or attractive. Fast or funny. We so want to stand out, to be enough.

As we strive we begin to feel, in an existential way, that we are, Brach says, "separate." Here we are, a self in here—and there everyone else is: out there. We feel alone and insecure. Which leads to a pervasive sense that something's wrong with our life. We can't understand: surely we aren't supposed to feel so alone. Everyone else can't feel as on their own as we do?

Pretty quickly, says Brach, that sense that "something's wrong" centers on the self. "We don't just ask ourselves, '*Is* something wrong?' Rather, it becomes an inner conviction that 'something's wrong with *me*.' That's the first conclusion that we make; it's the primal belief."

I'm intrigued.

I want to find out how this unconscious lack of self-acceptance fuels the negative floating brain and sabotages our efforts in mindfulness, meditation, and healing.

I reach out to Brach. When we speak by phone she explains to me that to some degree or another we all experience the emotional paper cuts of our culture of criticism, of our societal propensity for shame and blame.

I think about this. We all know the sinking feeling that comes with childhood admonishments over spilled milk, the math we didn't understand, the grade we didn't get. The clutch in the gut when no one picks us for dodgeball or asks us to the prom or the day our best friend dumps us for a new one and blabs our deepest secret in the exchange.

From *The Karate Kid* to *A Christmas Story*, Hollywood has made an industry of films in which the plot spins on such moments of childhood humiliation. Somewhere in the mix of whatever encouragement, support, and love we receive, there is a healthy dose of you-are-less-than.

I think, too, about the ACE studies. Over 60 percent of us have experienced at least one significant adverse childhood experience. Forty percent of us have experienced at least two. Whether our own ACE was a parent who wasn't there for us, or a parent who suffered from depression or alcoholism, or an adult in our lives who was at times emotionally cruel, we carry those stressful experiences, intermingled with whatever feelings of a loss of self-worth they engendered, into our lives now.

Brach believes we internalize this interior voice of criticism, carrying it with us into our criticism experiences both large and small, administering self-blame for everything including the cold we caught, the diagnosis we got, the ten pounds we gained, the fact that we didn't achieve what we thought we would in our career by the age of forty.

The more trauma we faced when we were young, Brach explains, or the more we were taught by our family or culture of origin to feel that there was something inherently wrong with us, "the more separate we feel."

To cover over our unmet need for unconditional love, we become ever more judgmental of ourselves, weaving ourselves into a deeper and tighter web of not-okay-ness. The process is so subtle we don't notice the disintegration of our self-view happening from the inside out.

Instead of applying love or kindness to ourselves when we need it, we turn into our worst best friend, the critic in the mirror. We stop being on our own side. And we begin to feel even more separate from the world around us.

Things evolve into a superficial view of the world: either we are doing well and things are going right and others take notice of us—or things are not going right and so we berate ourselves. Because things rarely seem right enough, we are usually unhappy with who we are, what we have, and what we've done.

"Believing that something is wrong with us is a deep and tenacious suffering," Brach tells me. Sometimes we project our feelings of unworthiness onto others and decide that whatever isn't going right has to be their fault. Yet even when we blame others, there's an undercurrent of "something is wrong with me." We figure if only we did more and did it better, we'd be okay.

The goal is, she says, "Not to be good to ourselves because we're afraid of what will happen if we aren't, but because we're really on our own side. Because we care about this life."

This turning on self gets in the way of so much joy, I suddenly think. If we've turned on ourselves, we can't love our world.

I am wondering something, however. "Isn't this intrinsically harder when we're facing a chronic health issue?" I ask Brach. "When we don't feel well on a physical level?"

I am surprised when Brach tells me that she is familiar with this struggle firsthand. She has a genetic connective tissue disorder that causes her to be injury prone and decreases her muscle strength. "Eight years ago I was starting to get sicker and sicker and I didn't want to acknowledge what was happening. I was getting more injuries and becoming weaker, but I wouldn't stop pushing myself. I had retreats to lead, and I didn't want to see myself as someone who was limited by illness."

Instead of resting as needed, Brach pushed herself to the point that on the eve of a major retreat she had been looking forward to teaching, she wound up spending the week in a hospital cardiac unit instead. It was a difficult time of self-reflection. "Not being able to control what's happening, and knowing that something is going wrong in our body, can make us feel we have to assign blame to something in order to regain our sense of control," she says. "The thought process goes like this: 'something is wrong and I have to assign blame in order to identify what can be fixed . . . if I can identify what is fixable, I can set out to fix it.' And this pretty quickly translates into deciding that we are to blame—'I don't take care of myself well, so of course I am sick.'" This, she says, makes us feel, for a time, that we have some sense of control. Even relief. We have, we tell ourselves, identified the problem.

Recently, Brach tells me, she tried speed walking even though she knew she shouldn't. She "completely screwed up" her knees. "I couldn't get up or down stairs for weeks. I am a terrible patient. And I found myself starting to hate myself for the fact that all my thoughts were becoming self-centered, and that I was so impatient and irritable with others. Here I was in an enormous amount of pain and I added more pain by not being able to stand myself for who I was when I was sick."

Struggling with a chronic illness can make it even harder to walk away from our feelings of self-dislike—even for an expert on the topic. And yet, says Brach, "It also reveals how acute and strong those feelings are, which can open the door to self-compassion."

AFTER WE HANG up the phone I don't have much time to process what she's said. I'm simply caught up in my rush of thinking about what needs to be done next—finish typing interview notes, send a few must-get-back-to-them e-mails, pick my kids up from the bus. Then a few errands to round up items Claire needs for a French project. I sigh. I don't know if I have the stamina today to run through the aisles of Target, Michael's, and Office Depot, but we must and we will. After dinner, I've got so much work left to do.

Then I hear it: the voice of my own self-lashing. It is as insidious as it is stealthy. Beneath the white noise of my chattering, thinking, planning mind, there is another darker whisper.

It is the voice that often sets in when I'm in physical pain or fatigued. *You're always tired, what the hell is the matter with you, you always have some impediment. You're robbing your kids by being so tired all the time. You never get enough work done; you're always behind. You'll never be who you dreamt you'd be. No wonder you got the lemon body that's always breaking down, that you can never count on—you deserve it.*

And then it hits me: this is my interior default setting. If things are not going swell—and how often are they going swell?—this is my brain's screensaver. This self-loathing gives birth to the Pain Channel. While I may not say the actual words, the effect is pretty much the same: *You loser.*

Suddenly I get it. How deep my sense of not-okay-ness is, like a scaffolding beneath everything I am and do.

And what is this default setting doing, I wonder, to my cells?

I recall the controversial work of a scientist who set out to document in photographs how human consciousness affects the molecules in water. In his book, *The Hidden Messages in Water,* Masuro Emoto found, he says, that when you wrap a glass of water with a piece of paper that says "love and gratitude" or "thank you," the water forms perfect, stunningly clear crystals. "I hate you," on the other hand, causes misshapen crystals to form.

Most particle physicists discount Emoto's work. But it's the image not the science that interests me here. I find the metaphorical idea behind his work intriguing. What is *You loser* doing to my molecules?

TRISH HAS GIVEN me a second piece of homework: to contemplate what my greatest stressors were when I was young, and to consider what early habits of mind I might have set in place when I met those stress points. Whether I was kind to myself in the face of long-ago adversity.

She's found that many of her mindfulness-based stress reduction, or MBSR, research participants have dealt with varied forms of childhood distress. Along the way, as Brach's work suggests, they've stopped being kind to themselves. For Trish's study participants, MBSR has proven quite useful in helping to bring a new perspective to the negative thoughts they have about themselves and others—and reverse the damaging floating brain that was set in motion in the earliest stages of their lives and in the worst of circumstances.

I don't have to think hard. Whenever my feelings back then were too much, when I just couldn't take anymore, I would imagine myself building a thick, red brick wall in my mind between what was happening around me and what was going on inside my own head.

I built that thick, red wall one brick at a time, carefully stacking each brick on top of the other so that no one could get past it. In my imagination I'd add mortar, place another brick on top, scrape off the excess, and add more bricks. I'd tell myself that on my side of the thick, red wall, I couldn't hear or feel anything. The adults around me could say what they wanted.

I filled my brain with my own mental churning—toward all the adults who'd let me down. *What do they know, why don't they all just shut up, what's wrong with them, didn't they even love him, if he were here he wouldn't put up with this*

It cut the feelings of missing my father, the ache I felt for him. It cut the ache of feeling that none of the grown-ups around me had my back. It obliterated everything: my mother's tears, the late-night conversations I'd overhear. The bitter blame. The criticisms.

I fed myself. I did my homework. I went to work right after school at the public library. I took care of what I could take care of, though it would be a stretch to say I took care of myself.

If I think about it clinically, yes, all of that probably constitutes childhood adversity. And those were surely less than productive habits of mind. But I just thought of it as one thing: lonely.

SUDDENLY, WITHOUT KNOWING how I got here, I'm pulling into the parking lot at the old, white mansion that houses Trish's office. I sit in the car for a moment or two until my eyes clear.

A FEW MINUTES later, upstairs, in Trish's office, I find myself relating all of it to her.

"I imagine I did a lot of damage to my young, neuroplastic brain," I confess to Trish now.

"Those angry tapes—and your red brick wall—served a critical purpose when you were young," she says, reading the look on my face. "They kept you alive. You didn't know a better way. You need to honor the role those tapes served for you when you were young; they were a tremendous coping mechanism in the face of untenable loss and confusion and fear. And they helped you to be less afraid in the face of your world coming down around you."

It's no surprise, she says, that I've continued to run angry and fearful thought tapes in my adult life—on topics and in situations now that are of course very different from those I faced when I was young. My health. My stamina. Even smaller irritations. Now, just as then, these negative thought cycles tend to surface when I feel I'm under stress—and I sure can't stop those tapes from playing when I try to sit still now.

"And yet now they really serve no good purpose," I confess. "I feel as if they're covering up my soul's inner language."

"Use a few describing words to name that language," Trish prompts. "Your soul's language?"

Three words rise up in me. "Joy. Creativity. Grief." I pause. "The mental churning, my racing thoughts cover up whatever joy and creativity might be there. I know the negative ruminating isn't good for me, but I can't shut those thought tapes down," I say. "And I don't feel justified in just sitting there, breathing, trying to harness an unquiet mind when there is so much else to be done."

"The first tenet of Buddhist teaching is that the mind is a waterfall," she says. "The awareness that it's rushing with thoughts is the first awakening." She pauses. "We first have to be aware that our mind is racing in order to begin to transform it. Often those of us who've been intellectualizing our feelings for so long are able to take note of how quickly our mind is racing once we watch for it. But for reasons having to do with our own history we may lack the self-love, the compassion for our own experience, to help us take the necessary and crucial second step."

That second step, she explains, is to have compassion for the way our mind works, for the thoughts we have, for the way in which our worry, angry resentments, jealousies, fears, and obsessive thoughts spin out of control. "Often when we have trouble meditating it's not due to a lack of awareness," Trish says, "but to a resistance to self-love."

Until our ability to be compassionate to ourselves becomes as strong as our awareness, well, then, we are not going to get very far when we sit down to try to quiet our mind.

"Our ability to be self-compassionate and forgive ourselves for having an unquiet mind, for having the thoughts and emotions we have, has to be as strong as our ability to be self-aware of how busy our mind is."

The Buddhists teach that the first arrow that strikes us is the experience we have. The second arrow is the shame we have about it and the blame we direct at ourselves. We find ourselves judging someone harshly or caught up in a torrent of tumbling grievances, and then we find ourselves judging our judging—blaming ourselves for being so unkind, for something we said or did, and asking, "How could I?"

The little things we get down on ourselves about—the lost piece of paper we put down somewhere but now can't find, the words we regret saying to the cable service person on the phone who has nothing to do with the highly annoying fact that our Internet is out for the third time that week—all seem, individually, to be so small and fleeting we don't realize they add up to one big negative state of mind.

If we've never turned a friendly eye on ourselves, we certainly won't recognize all this self-judging for what it is. We have no point of comparison. We just know it feels really bad to be in our own skin.

And that's where the part about childhood trauma makes things even trickier. When our world blows apart at a very young age, when we have to deal with adversity we don't understand and can't defend ourselves against, when there are no grown-ups to help us process what went wrong or offer us unconditional love, or to help us decode our feelings of loss and unworthiness when we need them most, we go into high-distress mode. We know on a biological level from epigenetic research on gene methylation that our PIN response gets stuck in the on position. We also know, on a psychological level, that when we are afraid our efforts at self-defense often devolve into churning out obsessive thoughts, spitting blame and anger at those who hurt us— all the while believing that we're rejected and unloved because there is something so fundamentally flawed with us that we've merely gotten what we deserved in the first place.

If we've been caught in that low-grade assumption of our own unworthiness from the time we were very young, if we can't relate to ourselves in a tender or sympathetic way because we never learned how, if we can't embrace our fears or flaws or pain the way we might if tending to a hurt child because no one ever modeled that for us, we have no way to cope but to just keep on churning angry thoughts and feeling unworthy. The lifelong pattern is set in place.

And so. If that is me, if that is the brain I have, how do I switch gears after so many years of negative mental churning? If I have been taking myself—and my negative brain—with me wherever I go for so many decades, how can I possibly set that brain down and create a new one?

Trish asks me to try the following at home, in the week before her MBSR training class begins:

1. When my tapes are spinning, take note of my mental speedometer. Notice where it is. One hundred fifty or ninety-five or twenty-two? Be aware.
2. See my mental churning as nothing more than a "habit of mind." It may or may not have relevance to the particular moment I'm actually in. If I'm ruminating over something that happened hours or years ago while folding laundry, it clearly doesn't.
3. Come up with a descriptive word or two to name my habit of mind. She asks me to offer up a few now. I come up with *mental spitting, fuming, churning.* She also suggests that I label my feelings: "This is anger," or "This is anxiety."

4. Ask myself if there is judging of my judging. In addition to the churning, am I judging myself for having my negative thoughts and feelings?
5. If so, actively place some words in my consciousness to be a balm to this second arrow, to lessen the sting of self-blaming.
6. Bring my focus to my breath as it is. Feel my breath filling my upper chest, my lungs, my abdomen. When my mind wanders, as it will, bring my focus back to my breath.

"WE ARE OFTEN stung by many self-judgments at the same time," Trish says. "Anger at someone, anger at ourselves for our own role in things, and anger at ourselves for how our mind is reacting to what happened." If we are judging ourselves, we have to step in and lessen that sting. She asks me to think of a phrase that might be my balm. Something along the lines of "Let it go," or "It's okay."

I can't think of a thing.

"What do you do for friends when they are going through a difficult time?" she asks.

"I make sure they know I love them."

"How?"

"I ask them to tell me all about it. I listen. I let them know that I love them and that I want to understand." I pause, searching for the right words. I say what comes to me: "I place my heart right next to them, as if it were a listening ear."

"Can you move in in that close and loving way for yourself?" she asks.

I'm silent. Tears well. The image in my mind is of a fire hose that's been stopped up with cement. Completely blocked. Some strong surge wants to come through but it can't. "I'm not so sure," I confess.

She suggests that I try placing my hand on my heart, or wherever I feel the sting. "Try saying just one word to yourself, whatever comes."

I put my hand to my heart. "Forgive me," I whisper. My heart thumps in my stomach.

She is quiet for a moment. Neither of us says anything. "It might help to try saying, 'Forgiven.'"

I am not sure why this one word hits me so hard. Why these tears from nowhere? At the thought of this one word?

Trish reads the question in my eyes. "If," she says softly, "after a lifetime of judging others as a survival mechanism, and judging yourself most harshly of all, one day you come to yourself with a loving heart, it may awaken old emotions, grief, that you don't yet understand." Yes, maybe it has to do with grief over what happened to me when I was twelve, or with a different kind of grief over the realization that I don't seem to care for myself. Or something else entirely.

I think she's going to tell me to try to delve into those emotions. Break them down. Unpack them. But she doesn't. "You needn't ask yourself what this experience means," she cautions. "It's not important to know anything about why those tears come up for you to practice mindfulness successfully.

"All that's needed is for you to stay close to your own experience," she says. "Be with whatever is happening. Feel it, experience it, but try not to entertain the question, 'What does forgiven mean?' Just go back to naming the experience. 'Here is grief. Here is doubt. Here is fear. Worry. Loss.' Parse out the narrative about why that feeling may be there. Catch the habits of your mind that are strong, name them, and drop in that piece of friendliness to yourself. Apply balm to the sting of self-judgment. Focus on working this new muscle over and over and over again."

She's seen in her research, she adds, that the practice of mindfulness retrains the brain toward a calmer place of wisdom and balance for those who've had a history of traumatic stress. This, in turn, allows deeper memories that are hard to deal with to arise for the first time. It becomes suddenly safe to deal with what we haven't dealt with before.

Hard-to-deal-with feelings or memories might arise—but when and if they do, she assures me, I'll be better able to see them for what they are and disarm the traumatic feelings and emotions that entrap me onto the distress highway. I'll be aware enough to separate out the here and now from the trauma of then, and deal with what I recall in a healthier way.

She suggests, meanwhile, that in an all-out effort on my own be-half, when I get home I write the word *forgiven* on sticky notes and paste them on the back of my hairbrush, on the bathroom mirror, in as many places as I can. Say "forgiven" to myself one hundred times a day if I have to.

Still, I can't help but wonder, exactly what do I need to be forgiven for?

WHEN I GET home I post sticky notes everywhere: the inside of a kitchen cupboard, the underside of the sun visor on the driver's side of my car. But I'm still curious about how the process of repeating a word will help me. If I am to name my feelings or apply a word to soothe myself one hundred times a day in order to feel better, I want to know why such a trick of the mind works. To really invest myself in the process, I want the science.

Certainly cultural wisdom tells us that talking out loud to a friend or a therapist, or writing in a journal, will make us feel better: when we put our loss, our fear, and fury into words, we heal. That's why if a friend is in pain, we encourage him or her to talk it out with us. If our children are hurt or afraid, we ask them to talk about how they feel and worry if they won't tell us.

It turns out, according to a team of neuroscientists at the University of California, Los Angeles, that these cultural instincts match up precisely with new scientific findings about how our brain functions. When we name our feelings we change the activity in our brain and bring ourselves into a calmer state of mind. We stop the negative floating brain in midflow.

Cognitive neuroscientists have long known that when they show subjects a picture of an angry or fearful face, the brain region known as the amygdala lights up. The amygdala, you might recall, is the same center that sparks the fight-or-flight process, raises the PIN response, and kicks the negative floating brain into fast and furious action. This heightened amygdala response holds true even if an individual views an angry facial expression subliminally—for such a split second he or she can't even recall having seen it a moment later.

Matthew Lieberman, PhD, UCLA professor of psychology and a leader in social cognitive neuroscience, along with his colleagues, decided to find out what might happen to an individual's amygdala response if he or she named the feelings associated with seeing those angry and fearful faces.

In the study, conducted at the brain-mapping center at UCLA, thirty subjects were shown faces that appeared angry or fearful. Below each face they saw one of either two words, such as *angry* or *fearful*. They were asked to choose which emotion applied to each expression they saw. Or, they saw two names, "Harry" and "Sally," and were asked to choose the gender-appropriate answer for each face. Meanwhile, Lieberman and his colleagues used functional magnetic resonance imaging (MRI) to study each participant's brain activity.

When participants attached the word *angry* to an angry face and labeled the feeling, researchers saw a decrease in their amygdala response. When participants simply attached a name, such as Harry, their amygdala response stayed fired up.

But something else happened that researchers found quite intriguing. When study subjects labeled the feeling associated with each face, another area of the brain, known as the right ventrolateral prefrontal cortex, became more active. This area, which sits just behind the forehead and eyes, is associated with thinking about emotional experiences in words, helping to process emotions, and helping us to change our behavioral response to them. Researchers are, frankly, still a little fuzzy about everything the right ventrolateral prefrontal cortex does, but two things are clear: it is the area responsible for helping us to name our emotions and, when it lights up, the amygdala-driven fight-or-flight response goes significantly down.

UCLA researchers wanted to investigate this one step further. They wanted to know whether labeling one's thoughts through practicing mindfulness meditation—saying, for instance, "I'm feeling angry right now" or "This is fear"—would also light up the right ventrolateral prefrontal cortex and turn down the amygdala alarm center response in the brain.

They scanned individuals' brains while they practiced mindfulness meditation and had them fill out fine-grained questionnaires afterward about how often they had mindfully labeled their feelings.

It turned out that the meditators who reported labeling their emotions the most by employing mindfulness also had the greatest activation in the right ventrolateral prefrontal cortex and this, in turn, decreased activity in the amygdala. In fact, the more mindful participants were in labeling their feelings with words, the less amygdala activation researchers saw.

The more we utilize the center of our brain that names feelings, the less stressed we feel by them.

That's pretty big news.

Lieberman likens the process of naming your feelings to hitting the brake when you're driving along and suddenly see a yellow light. "By putting your feelings into words," he says, "it's as if you're hitting the brakes on your emotional responses."

You feel less angry, less sad, less afraid.

Lieberman's work may also help, in part, to explain why talk therapy has been found to be as effective as medication for moderate depression; that patients who undergo talk therapy show brain pattern changes similar to those seen in people taking antidepressants; and that talk therapy is more effective long-term for seasonal affective disorder than the traditional treatment, light therapy, alone.

Lieberman's research likewise suggests to us that one neurocognitive mechanism that might explain how meditation improves health outcomes is the decreased amygdala response that occurs when we label negative events. That, in turn, decreases the level of stress hormones and inflammatory cytokines rushing through the body.

One other interesting finding from the study also jumps out at me.

Lieberman believes that this newly understood right ventrolateral prefrontal cortex may be particularly affected by what happens during our preteen and teenage years. This area of the brain undergoes much of its crucial development during that time. It may be, he hypothe-sizes, that a young person's emotional interactions with family and friends shape the strength of this brain region's response and impact it for life—depending on how healthy his or her emotional environ-ment was. If a teen is coming of age in an emotionally healthy envi-ronment, this area of the brain should be strong and resilient. If his or her environment is less stable, this area of the brain may be less ca-pable of ameliorating the amygdala response.

I think about this, in the context of what we know about the legacy of adverse childhood experiences, or ACEs. It would seem that if one had little help or support during traumatic preteen or teen years, it may be harder later in life to recognize one's emotions for what they are, name them, voice them, and feel better—and heal from tiny hurts and large ones. The right ventrolateral prefrontal cortex's processing abilities might be compromised for life.

We don't have any studies on this yet. We don't know if kids with significant ACE scores have more trouble when they grow up being mindful, naming their feelings, or being kind to themselves in the face of their emotional reactivity.

But I suspect that even though the hard science on this is still out-standing, we already know the answer.

I think I do.

Playing Catch with Thoughts in Midair

The next morning Zen drops me off to pick up my car, which we dropped off the night before for a new timing belt and an oil change. We wave good-bye in a rush. He has a nine a.m. meeting in Washington. I am headed to northern Virginia to do an interview with an expert in muscle tension and mood. It has been drizzling all morning, and the October sky is not promising, which means traffic will be an issue.

I head into our mechanic's office, pay the bill, pick up the key.

I get in the car. Someone on his staff has left his Coke can in one of the drink holders. And a few grease-oozing wadded-up Pizza Boli's napkins in the other one. I touch the steering wheel. Greasy. Sticky. I take a deep breath. When I am in a hurry and things around me are messy and dirty—well, that's not a good combination. So often the universe serves the two up at the same time. Like pizza and Coke.

How could they leave all their crud in my car?

You would think . . . A deep reverberation of irritation travels through my chest—all the way to my abdomen. It doesn't feel good.

I pause. I draw upon my new trick, trying it again, like a toddler trying out the delicious feeling of mashing a banana for the second and third time. *This is frustration! Thinking! Judging!*

Better.

I turn on the engine. I punch the radio to listen to NPR as a way to distract me from my frustration and wait for navigation to come on so I can input the address of the office building where I'm meeting my expert in an hour.

The radio doesn't come on.

No navigation.

I wait.

A blank screen. A silent radio.

I turn the car off. I turn it back on. Nothing.

We bought this car used and one of the reasons we bought it was this: the car was a phenomenal price and though we were not shopping with the criteria of having navigation, we do live a three-city life and the idea of having a cheat system to get us from here to there with fewer hours at the computer on MapQuest and fewer wrong turns suddenly seemed . . . essential. Right or wrong, I've come to rely on it to make my life work given the fact that I am directionally challenged and so is Zen.

I go back in to talk to the owner of the mechanic shop, who is a lovely guy; he has kept each of our cars running beautifully for the eleven-plus years we eke out of each vehicle.

"L!" I tell him the navigation is out. "I have to be on the other side of DC in an hour!" I say.

In the twenty years he's worked on our cars, he's never heard me raise my voice. His eyebrows go up. "Let's see what's going on," he says.

I turn to open the door of the shop and forget how fast his door swings open, and how slowly my foot moves. The door scuffs over the top of my sandal and whacks into the right side of my left toe. Pain broadcasts through nerve endings I thought I no longer had. I stand there for a moment, hoping my face is not turning bright red.

He gets in the car and starts pushing a few buttons. "Huh," I hear him say as I hobble toward him. "When we put in the new timing belt we must have reset everything and it didn't reboot."

I can't speak. I'm in pain. I'm annoyed. I'm late. I fish out the instruction book that I keep in the glove compartment. I can't believe it. Here I am, standing by my car with my mechanic, reading the car manual with him. As he leafs through pages and punches buttons I am seething. Not at him, per se, but at the situation.

My emotions are coming on so fast I can't even consider any other options except the dark side.

How the hell am I going to find the office building where I'm doing my interview? I have to leave! My brain is sledding on ice down the mountain. *I'll be late. I'll miss my appointment. Traffic will be backed up on the beltway in the rain.* My foot throbs. I look down. My left toe is bright red, the toenail purple. *I'm such a klutz! My navigation breaks. My body breaks down. Everything always breaks! My whole life is broken!*

In less than a minute my entire view from within has shifted one hundred eighty degrees.

THIS DOESN'T FEEL like being late, or getting lost, or something mechanical breaking. It feels like something bigger.

L is punching in more numbers. We've found the reset code for my radio. The fifth time we plug it in, it works.

But navigation still isn't working.

"It just needs half an hour before it will reboot," he says. "If it doesn't come on by tonight, call me and we'll look at it again in the morning."

"Thanks," I say, as if I am really standing here, right in front of him, talking, though I am actually racing along with the feelings of fury and frustration and pain charging through my body, like a dog that can't stop chasing a car.

He gives a small, silent wave as I get in my car and buckle up.

As I drive off I realize something else. My gas tank is on empty. I'd forgotten that I had no gas. I pull into the station, fill up, then get back into the driver's seat to find my phone. The smell of gas permeates the car. I must have stepped in a puddle of gasoline. The smell is nauseating. *I have no idea where I'm going, and I am going to be late, and I am going to get to my interview stinking like gasoline, and that is going to be just so . . . like Donna.*

I roll down the window for air and pull down the windshield's sun visor to shield me from the sun's glare. Just then, a small breeze enters the car. Something on the underside of the sun visor flutters. I stare at it for a minute before I realize it is the same sticky note that I put there, days ago, and promptly forgot about. I blink as I read what it says: *Forgiven.*

My mind begins to swim back to me.

I check my internal speedometer: 220. *You're not me,* I say to my racing Indie 500 thoughts. *I am not my thoughts.*

Go back to the plan.

First step, recognize where you are. *This doesn't feel good. I am not enjoying this.*

Name the feeling. *Here is self-loathing. Thinking! Worrying!*

What next? my brain asks me, with the desperation of a blindfolded prisoner walking the plank.

I hear Trish's voice in my mind, "Apply balm to the sting."

The gas pump clicks off. I replace the nozzle. "Forgiven," I say out loud, putting my hand to my chest so subtly I hope anyone else who happens to be pumping gas might think I'm just scratching an itch. I screw in my gas tank cap.

The tug of tears again, as if with some old ache.

Forgiven. For worrying. For feeling mad. For being ill. For being stupid. Forgiven for what I don't understand; whatever makes my heart brim in my chest at the very mention of the word.

I feel the grip, the clutch, in my body begin to release. I remember Trish coaching me, "Say it one hundred times a day if you have to." So I do. I say it again. "Forgiven." The path to mindfulness comes rushing back to me. Something clicks. *Bring your focus to your breath.* I fill my upper chest, my lungs, and my belly with breath. Hold it there for a moment. Let it go. I can almost hear the screaming meemies feeling escaping me, as if my feelings were air escaping a helium balloon.

When we are mindful, when we simply watch our thoughts and sensations come and go, and note that our mental spitting just doesn't match up to what's really happening, right now, we can step in and intercede. When we label our habits of mind and apply balm to the sting, we get to come back into the present, untainted by our worst imaginings. We get to come back to who we really are. And what we really feel. Mindfulness holds up a mirror that shows us what's really happening, undistorted, so we can respond with a rational mind.

And the act of just naming our feelings—the science now tells us—provides that pause for us.

My mind opens a little more, expanding toward a wide-angle view.

The computer in the car will reboot later; if not, I will take it back to the shop. I won't be late if I call ahead to my interview and get directions the old-fashioned way. The pain in my toe is already easing. I can clean the soles of my sandals with my water bottle and keep the window down until the smell of gasoline dissipates.

Yes, there is deeper stuff, beneath the surface pain. When I drill down, I can feel it all hovering there. That ache. But for here and now, everything is really nowhere near as bad as it seems.

I fall back, hard, to the lesson I keep forgetting. I have assumed, all my life, that I am my feelings. That if my spinning thoughts keep cycling back, then they are real. If my feelings and I are one, then they must be real because I am real, right? We are as real as the rain spattering my windshield, and the situation is a crisis at hand—*just because it feels like one.*

But some blessed part of me remembers: this is the primary illusion. We don't have to react to the thoughts and feelings inside our mind as if they are true. They are emotions that will vary and change through the hours or days—as unpredictable as the internal weather. Another front is always coming in. Another front is always moving out.

I have choices in how I see them. I have my view from within.

There are steps I can take when the speedometer and *vroom* revving inside my skull don't match up with the milder reality of what's going on around me.

I have the first necessary pieces of equipment to hang on my tool belt, to help me build the framework for joy, and set a positive feedback loop in motion.

I think of a story a friend once shared about a meditation newbie who was going up on an elevator to her room at a meditation retreat, rushing, late to check in, not sure she should even be taking the time to go away when she was so behind at work. When the elevator got to her floor, the door wouldn't open. She pressed the open-door button over and over but still nothing happened. She started cursing. This sort of thing always happened to her; nothing ever went her way, and here she was stuck on the stupid elevator—of course she would be the one! She was furiously punching the button hard for the twentieth time when she heard a voice behind her, "Ellen, the door opens on *this* side."

All she had to do was turn around. The doors were wide open.

Her perception of her situation was false. Therefore her reaction had to be false as well.

I dial the number for the expert I'm headed to interview, and it turns out the directions to get to her office are quite simple. I write them down and start the car.

· 10 ·

So How Did We Get This Way?

Until now I've been looking at our proclivity to tune into the Pain Channel through a personal lens. But much of our threat reactivity isn't in the least bit specific to our personal genetics or experience. To some extent, no matter our story, we're all in the same boat, paddling upriver, against the swift current of our own thinking. Our individual biology is only one reason why we're so predictably reactive to the potential threats around us. We are also up against hundreds of thousands of years of evolutionary biology: veering toward the negative is a trait we share with all seven billion *Homo sapiens* alive today because of the way we humans evolved.

No one knows more about this than neurospychologist Rick Hanson, PhD, cofounder of the Wellspring Institute for Neuroscience and Contemplative Wisdom and author of *Buddha's Brain: The Practical Neuroscience of Happiness, Love & Wisdom.*

Hanson writes and talks extensively about the complexity of the brain and why, in order to ensure our evolutionary advantage, the brain keeps us so closely attuned to what's bad or potentially wrong in our lives.

It may help, first, to appreciate what a stunningly busy place the brain is. In the time it takes for you to read this sentence—about one breath cycle—a quadrillion-plus messages will course through your head, with signals crossing the brain in a tenth or even a hundredth of a second.

All our thinking, worries, and hopes enter our conscious thought courtesy of the hectic traffic zooming between 1.1 trillion brain cells and one hundred billion gray matter neurons—as they fire away in our brain sending signals to other neurons. Each neuron connects with about five thousand other neurons, meaning about five hundred trillion synapses are constantly making connections as the brain moves information around the way the heart moves our blood around.

To accomplish all this, our brain utilizes 20 to 25 percent of our body's blood flow and oxygen at any given moment.

Research tells us that much more of this brain activity, oxygen, and blood flow is dedicated to the service of our negative thoughts, to fear and rumination, rather than to positive ones.

Why are our brains hardwired this way?

It's survival of the fittest, learned at Mother Nature's knee. When we were still lighting fires, living in caves, and hunting wild boar, the caveman whose brain constantly scanned his immediate surroundings for every possible threat had a leg up on the fellow who wasn't as clued into what might go wrong. If some part of your brain wasn't autosearching the night for the rustle of a saber-toothed tiger in the bushes, or ruminating with suspicion that the wandering caveman who joined your clan might put a spear in your back, your chances of being dead by morning went up.

Noticing the good got you very little, in evolutionary currency. Yes, the snow shimmering on trees or the sight of birds in midflight might be beautiful, but what did Mother Nature care about that? If your brain was occupied with picking beautiful wildflowers, you might miss the saber-toothed cat stalking you. End of your gene pool.

"For millions of years, fear and worry gave us the competitive edge," says Hanson. That's why in the amygdala, the "alarm center" in the brain, two-thirds of the cells are dedicated processors for negative or potentially negative information. This is the part of the brain that dates back all the way to our reptilian predecessors, which is why it's often referred to as the "lizard brain." It differs from the prefrontal cortex, the area of the brain that makes us stop, think, and reconsider whatever situation we find ourselves in. The prefrontal cortex helps us to analyze, plan—and look before we leap. But it takes its time making decisions. The amygdala, on the other hand, scans our environment, moment to moment, to see what's a threat, and makes a superfast snap judgment as to whether we should react with anxiety and fear. It's hardwired to focus on negative information and react to it intensely. The pressing question for the amygdala is "Am I safe?"

The amygdala and the hippocampus, the areas of the brain that process visual spatial memory and put our memories in varied contexts, such as good or bad, rapidly flag anything even remotely negative, storing it away for future reference.

If the memory is bad, the amygdala stores it and underscores it so that it can be retrieved on a fast track of rapid-fire neurons the next time a similar situation occurs. That way, when our caveman ancestor heard a rustling of leaves in the bushes, he remembered, in a flash, that this could mean a man-eating tiger in the vicinity and imminent death.

There is a memorable saying, coined by Hanson, that our brain is like Velcro for negative events, and Teflon for positive ones.

Every day, we all face an inner battle to try to balance our brain's natural, deeply ingrained evolutionary-based tendency to see what Hanson refers to as "paper tigers" everywhere. We have evolved to mistakenly assume, he explains, that there is a tiger in the bushes ten thousand times for every time there may be one—in order to avoid making a life-or-death mistake even once.

Not surprisingly, the level of our ingrained threat reactivity is intensified by our own unique life history. If we routinely had tigers jumping out of bushes when we were growing up—the alcoholic or bipolar parent, the sudden death of someone we loved—our brains will become all the more threat fearful and reactive. If our bushes turned out not to have a single tiger in them, we will respond to the world around us with less of a hair trigger.

The brain Velcro-ing to bad things is one more reason why the negative memories that accompany traumatic scenes from our childhood can still seem so real decades later. They replay in Technicolor detail, as if our mind had taken a video and filed it away. On the other hand, it's hard to recall the dozens of intimate family nights at the dinner table playing Uno, unless it was interrupted by an unforgettable moment, like, say, the birthday dinner when we finally got that red Schwinn racing bike.

Let's imagine a child who, as we all do, shares the biological evolutionary predisposition to see paper tigers everywhere. Now let's say she's also had, as 40 percent of us have, two or more especially stressful adverse childhood experiences, or ACEs, which, as discussed in earlier chapters, lead to increased gene methylation, causing her PIN response to become stuck in the full-throttle position. Let's say, too, that she's had her share of chronic stress as an adult. She's divorced, has chronic health problems, and she recently lost her job.

If we look around us or just in the mirror, most of us will have to admit that's not such an unusual or hypothetical "she" or "he."

All too often, it's the human condition.

As we engage in more and more habitually negative thoughts, rehearsing particular losses or painful memories, making assumptions that the world and the people in it are untrustworthy and out to get us, we cause groups of neurons to fire together. These firings wire new neural structures in our brain, leaving deep neurological grooves and lasting imprints that influence us to keep on having similar negative thoughts in the same direction long into the future. Positron emission tomography (PET) scans of the brain show that the more we ruminate and spin stories and relive bad memories, or beat up on ourselves or others, the more we reinforce the synapses associated with those negative thought patterns in our brain matter, and the more those synapses begin to fire by habit.

Our habits of mind direct the development of our neural structure much like a river cutting its way across a mountain terrain, says Hanson. The more we direct the river in one direction, the deeper and wider cuts it makes in the rock's surface, until the water flows ever more quickly and easily in one direction. Suddenly, our worst habits of mind come to us more frequently, effortlessly, unbidden—in a torrent.

Our brain begins to trigger those thoughts for us—before we even think them—redirecting our thinking down a negative track. The more those synapses habitually fire, the more negative thoughts we think. The more negative thoughts we think, the more those synapses habitually fire. The negative feedback cycle spins on.

This sounds dreadful—and it feels dreadful.

But the fact that the brain is so neuroplastic—that we can sculpt its structure with our mental activity—is very, very good news. It gives us the opportunity to intervene inside the black box of the brain and choose whether to lay down negative tracks or positive ones.

Joseph LeDoux, a professor of neuroscience and psychology at New York University, once said, "Much of who we are is based on memories learned through personal experience. . . . In fact, genes and experience, or nature and nurture, are, in the end, not different things, but different ways of doing the same thing—*wiring the synapses of our brain.* In many ways, the self is synaptic." Everything we think and feel and keep thinking and feeling creates, deep within, the brain we have and will have.

The habit of mind becomes us; we become the habit of mind. Gandhi said it thus: "Your beliefs become your thoughts. Your thoughts become your words. Your words become your actions. Your actions become your habits. Your habits become your values. Your values become your destiny."

States of joy and contentment not only create healthier neural circuitry patterns, they have an added benefit. They change the brain—and our habits of mind. They fire up the left frontal region of the brain that provides us with a profound feeling of well-being. The more we experience these states, the more easily and quickly we're able to calm ourselves or feel positive at will, and enter that state of feeling that all will be okay, all will be right with the world—despite what might be going on around us. The more we change what's happening in the mind, the more we change the brain, and the more we change the brain, the more we change what's happening in the mind.

Just to level the playing field, then, we have to shift our own internal balance toward being positive. As Hanson puts it, "We need to help ourselves see the world clearly, not ignoring the actual threats that are out there, but waking up from the paranoid trance that thinks it's always Threat Level Orange."

And that is going to require a bit of work.

Yet it can be done. The principal activity of the brain, Hanson reassures us, is to "make changes in itself." The residue of our minute-by-minute conscious experience continually shifts into our neural structure. We can, he says, begin to engage in "reverse engineering," incrementally altering the "expression of strips of atoms inside our own molecules"—creating "improved gene expression in the portion of our DNA that down regulates the stress response."

In the past twenty years, says Hanson, our knowledge about the brain has doubled. And this historically unprecedented knowledge about how our psychological state impacts our cells gives us a historically unprecedented opportunity.

We can—all of us—shift the neural substrate inside the black box of the brain and build those neural substrates out in increasingly skillful ways until we reach an "optimal state of functioning."

"For those among us who have experienced our share of ACEs," says Hanson, "it's all the more important to 'support our physiology' through good health practices—including exercising and eating right—and to engage in the work of mental retraining."

Until we get back on the Life Channel.

· 11 ·

Breath Works

A few days after my scene in the car, I start Trish's MBSR class, where, for the next eight weeks, I will work with a group of eleven other students who hope to change their way of being in and reacting to the world around them.

Most of the work I've done so far has been on the fly—trying to bring Trish's mindfulness and meditation suggestions into my daily life as best I can. But now, I'll be sitting still in a quiet room, attempting to meditate the way Saron's meditators do—focusing on quieting my mind for half hour or even hour-long stretches at a time. Trying to keep my mind on my breath, and coming back to the breath when my mind wanders away.

Trish begins by walking us through a set of exercises to help us settle into being present before we begin our mindful breathing.

The first step is to anchor ourselves, physically, in the here and now.

Trish asks us to notice our thighs and back touching the chair. "Drop in the question," she says. "How am I feeling right now?"

Now that's an emotional oxymoron. My body screams at me all day: twisting stomach with shooting pains, numb feet, headache, brain fog, fingers scratching, scratching at my eczema rash, back spasms. Flu-deep fatigue I never talk about to anyone. It is what it is. I never ask myself the question "How am I feeling right now?" because I don't care to hear the response my body will fire back at me.

"Even if you don't like what you find that's okay," Trish interjects. "Just move in close and apply a little friendliness. If your back or shoulder or knee hurts, get in close and meet any discomfort or pain with a sense of kindness."

I give it a try. I focus on the fatigue contracting my brain like a headache that never goes away. I hate this foggy, dopey fatigue. I move in close, anyway. *Ache. Fog. Tired. So tired.*

"Ask yourself, 'What else am I feeling right now?' Move in a little closer," Trish says. "And be friendly to whatever your experience is."

I try, moving in a little closer like a camera panning in.

The familiar fog sits there, like a veil that won't part.

But there is also something else. Sitting in my brain, beneath the headache, the fatigue, the self-flagellation over the fatigue.

Sadness.

I'm startled. I know I sometimes get anxious. Worried. Frenzied. Tired. Frustrated. Overwhelmed. Sometimes I have to lie down. A lot of times I have to lie down.

But I do not think of myself as being sad.

Still, I feel it lying there, intractable. As if some dormant creature is waking up and is slowly chewing its way along my brain synapses.

And noticing it for the first time seems to make it momentarily worse. Like that swollen feeling around your brain a second before you realize you're about to cry.

Such sadness. How long has it been there? And what do I do with it?

THE PROBLEM WITH getting so quiet is that noisy things come up. How do you change your view from within when what's there feels like a heavy, immovable force?

"If you're getting lost in a negative emotion, take in a deep breath and let out a mindful sigh," Trish says, walking us through the three mindful sighs technique. We all take in a collective deep "three-part" breath, breathing deeply through the nose, first into the lower belly, then the stomach, then the chest—as if inhaling into three separate balloons. Then letting it out, every last bit of air, until our belly collapses back into the spine. Everywhere around me I hear long, enormous exhales. Suddenly the room is full of the weight of love gone amiss, careers that didn't pan out, health anxieties, angst for children grown and growing.

It helps to let the sound out. It helps to know I'm not alone. The ache sits there, but the emotion that surrounds it starts to dissipate. *No need to follow it.*

We sigh again. Our personal stories aside, we are all up against our shared evolutionary biology: the hardwired compulsion to worry and beware—or be eaten alive. For thousands of years, the most worried ruminators in our evolutionary past were the ones who lived to dominate our gene pool.

I recall hearing the Venerable Khandro Rinpoche—one of only a handful of female Tibetan teachers and the only female teacher to have come to the West to teach—give a talk in which she provided a reassuring vignette. She remembers, she says, once complaining to her teacher, "These thoughts just won't cease." And her teacher turning around and saying, "They will when you die. A corpse has no thoughts. Get on with it." Thoughts, Rinpoche teaches, are "a very natural expression of a very vivid mind." A mind, that is, that is very much alive. She sometimes jokes to her students, "Don't worry, if you set down your thoughts for fifteen minutes to meditate, all those thoughts will still be waiting for you when you stop meditating."

Sometimes when I'm trying to quiet my brain noise I feel a compulsion to work through each thought—as if once I've gone through my crowded mind and addressed each problem or plan or resentment or fear, I'll be thought-free. But the truth is I'll never think it all through. As any of us who try to meditate know all too well, our thoughts aren't going anywhere. If you can stave them off for fifteen minutes or even fifteen seconds by focusing on the breath, well, that's a coup. They'll still be right there, waiting for you the second you're finished.

If our thoughts are especially intrusive, Trish tells us, we can try counting one on the in breath, then letting out a long, silent *ahhh* on the out breath. Count two on the next in breath, with a silent *ahhh* on the out breath. If we work our way up to ten breaths without being interrupted by thoughts, we can start again at one. If we get lost, come back and start at one again.

I give it a go. Three breaths. That's how far I get.

"Research tells us that if we can simply stay focused on the breath for twelve seconds, our brain begins to enter a state of concentration," Trish tells the class, her voice soft, encouraging. "And we build up tracks in our brain that help us to return to that state of concentration more easily the next time."

I do find this reassuring. Twelve seconds. The magic number. About how long it takes to take three deep breaths in and out. This I think I can do. After all, I have just done it. I can do it again.

Except that my legs, which have been falling asleep despite my rubbing and shaking them, are sending sharp pins and needle pricks all the way to my brain. I move in close. "This too is okay," I say to my shins, my ankles, and my toes, which feel as if sparklers are igniting beneath my skin. To my brain. To my fatigue. To the sadness beneath the fatigue. *It's okay if you can't stay focused on your breathing. It's okay if you feel heavy inside and don't know why. It's okay if your not-so-great legs sometimes turn to rubber. This too is all right.*

And then it hits me. How I am not beating myself up for the fact that my legs are not like other people's legs. Even though I have been a poor student of the breath, I am present, with my experience, and something inside feels *okay* with what I'm experiencing, with my feelings, my fatigue, my numb legs. And that okayness with my disappointing body is something entirely new.

· · ·

I'M INTRIGUED BY how much the act of heavily sighing out loud helps me to move into a deeper state of concentration and relaxation. So when I get home I read up on a bit of recent research. It turns out mood-related "sound signatures" help us to release the stress and tension we unwittingly hold tight in different places in our bodies.

It's pretty interesting. When we're happy we laugh. When we're sad we cry. When we're afraid we belt out a scream. But there are so many emotions between grief and gladness, between loss and fright. Most of life lies in between those bigger sounds. With what sounds do we release those feelings—and when?

Most of us avoid sighing for fear of being thought martyrish. But sighing, experts say, is a great way to off-gas emotions: the frustrations and ruminations and hurts and fears that don't otherwise get released. Why? It helps to kick in the parasympathetic nervous system and calm us down.

I think of my mother—after she lost my dad and found herself with four teenagers to raise alone, sighing became her signature sound. She sighed as she drove, talked, looked through cupboards in the kitchen. Sighing, sighing, until the sighs sounded like buzzing insects I wanted to distance myself from. Now I realize that her sighs were self-soothing, quieting her own PIN response, helping her to off-gas, at least a little, the negative energy of her own floating brain.

Preparing to sigh also forces us to take in a slightly deeper breath than we otherwise might. Most of us are chest breathers—we rarely bring air to our lower lungs. When we do a three-part inhalation, or simply prepare to sigh because we're fed up with someone or something, we draw a deeper breath in, which also helps to quiet the sympathetic nervous system.

Some Tibetan teachers, such as Tsoknyi Rinpoche, the Tibetan head of monasteries and nunneries in Tibet and Nepal, who is particularly interested in the intersection between ancient Tibetan Buddhist tradition and neuroscience, and how meditation practice can benefit us normal folk in our everyday lives, teach mindful sighs as three very rapid exhales. Cliff Saron recently sent me a talk that Tsoknyi Rinpoche gave in which he meditated with a group of neuroscientists at a conference, practicing this technique. Take a big, three-part deep breath in, inhaling as much as you can. Hold that inhalation for a few seconds, then exhale very hard and loud and rapidly: *haaaaaaaaaaaaaaaaaa*. A loud, vehement extra-fast mammoth exhale, letting it all out. Pain. Fear. Mental demons.

When we do this, says Rinpoche, "the fixation goes away." Instead, we feel "clarity, fearlessness, openness."

It works. I've tried it. It leaves me with that sudden clearheaded feeling I get for a split second after I sneeze. For a millisecond I can't recall what I was worrying about before the sneeze distracted my entire body. Only the three rapid exhale technique's effects last a little longer and can be done at will.

IN MY READING I come across another breath exercise, called "alternate nostril breathing." It's very simple. And I find it very powerful. We bring our thumb to the right side of our nose and our ring finger to the left side—making a sort of U-shaped peace sign with our pointer and middle fingers down against our palm and then thumb, leaving our ring finger and pinky pointing up. Then we place our thumb on the right side of our nose and close off our right nostril. Inhale through the left. Then we close our left nostril with our ring finger and slowly exhale and inhale through the right nostril. Then we close off the right nostril with our thumb . . . and repeat the sequence eight times on each side.

When I finish I give a little laugh to myself. Get this, I tell myself: I just made it to eight uninterrupted breaths. It took so much concentration to follow the instructions I really didn't have a choice.

THAT AFTERNOON I try combining alternate nostril breathing with deep three-part inhalations and exhalations at home, over my computer, when fatigue and cloudy-headedness threaten to send me for a lie-down I don't have time for. I decide to experiment: the bus comes in twenty-five minutes. I have four pretty important e-mails to send before I meet the bus and head out for the after-school rush around. This breath exercise will take me four minutes. Lying down is never that simple.

Four minutes later my brain feels buzzy—in a good way. And I have twenty-one minutes to spare.

THE NEXT MORNING, Saturday, I wake up determined to really, truly meditate—or what meditators refer to in shorthand as "sit"—before the day gets away from me. As usual, I am afraid of trying and failing. At least if I fail at night I have an excuse—I fell asleep.

I think of what Trish says. The most important thing is not how long we are able to stay wedded to the breath, but that when we notice we're not with the breath we catch ourselves, and then come back to it. "If we never wandered from the breath, we wouldn't reap the benefits of making new pathways in the brain," she says. "Every time our mind wanders it's a new opportunity to create those new synapses, which in turn will make it easier to stay with the breath over time."

I set the timer for fifteen minutes and sit cross-legged, slightly braced by the bed's headboard, on a stack of pillows so high I can wiggle my legs every few minutes to keep my nerves in my legs alert. Each time a worried thought comes I try to veer back to the breath. And come they do, nonstop, like soldiers, cannon fodder for the brain. One after the other. Planning the schedule for tomorrow. Wondering why the dog threw up again. Gas is so expensive. I have to call my mother back. How am I going to finish my deadline for tomorrow? It's not possible! I wish my friend with multiple sclerosis were feeling better. I worry about her. Why is the dog throwing up so much?

To calm myself a little I use a "relaxing breath" exercise that's a little different from three mindful sighs; a friend of mine sent it to me last week. My friend says her husband, who suffers from anxiety attacks and used to breathe into a brown paper bag to calm himself down when one struck, now uses this instead. I want to see if the technique, developed by Andrew Weil, MD, works for me, too. I place the tip of my tongue against my upper row of teeth, breathe in through my nose to the count of four, hold my breath to the count of seven, then exhale through my mouth to the count of eight, making a loud, whooshing sound. You do this through four cycles, working your way up to eight over time.

It is still early morning. I hear the birds singing in the tree outside my window as I inhale. Exhale. I hear Claire pad softly into my room. I sense her standing there, then leaving. Then she comes back in again, the door creaking as she softly closes it, as if I might not hear. Slowly, even as I take in the sounds around me, my own sense of being here, of being alive, seems to grow. Magnify. My eyes are so heavy with this new, sweet moment of openness that I can't yet lift my lids. The space I feel inside widens. I'm like a low-flying kite, skimming along the ground. I don't want to leave the moment. Even as I imagine my daughter staring at her mom sitting cross-legged against the damask headboard.

I feel her creep up onto the bed. Ashlie has taken advantage of the open door and come in with her. She jumps up, curling in the perfect triangle made by my legs. Claire slips her head into my lap, too, resting her head half on my knee, half on the puppy.

Mother, daughter, rescue pup. The girls. They both seem to sense the quiet of the moment and we slip further into it together. I slide one hand onto Claire's head and my other palm falls on the dog's soft fur.

Ten minutes pass. Breath. Daughter. Dog. Love.

The timer goes off. For the first time, I feel it's way too soon to stop.

Claire lifts her head. "Mom, can we walk the dog?"

· 12 ·

The Compassion Cure

One of the foremost researchers studying the benefits of loving-kindness, or compassion, meditation is Dr. Charles Raison, until recently codirector of the Emory Collaborative for Contemplative Studies and clinical director of the Emory University Mind-Body Program, and now the Barry and Janet Lang Associate Professor of Integrative Mental Health at the University of Arizona. On any given day you might find nineteen-year-old college sophomores—or the Dalai Lama encircled by his maroon–and-gold-robed monks—practicing compassion meditation in Raison's lab, allowing Raison and his colleagues to scrutinize changes in their stress hormones, inflammatory markers, and immune function.

Loving-kindness is an ancient practice that is said to have originated with the Buddha. The story goes that his followers were once meditating in the forest when they encountered frightening tree spirits. The Buddha taught them this practice as an antidote to fear.

Loving-kindness is quite a different practice from mindful breathing, which calms the mind by helping us to be aware of our thoughts, then let our future planning, our worry, our regret go, and return to the breath.

Loving-kindness involves repeating specific phrases that send a series of loving thoughts to ourselves, those we love, those we barely know, those we find difficult to deal with, and, finally, all beings everywhere.

The Dalai Lama and his monks are well-known for their practice of compassion meditation in a Tibetan tradition known as Lojong mind training. In Lojong mind training, which seeks to refine and purify one's motivations and attitudes, meditators practice to rid their mind of the undesired mental habits that cause suffering. One of the fifty-nine slogans that inform the practice is "Be grateful to everyone."

Compassion meditation uses a cognitive, analytic approach to challenge our unexamined thoughts and emotions toward other people, with the long-term goal of helping us to develop more altruistic emotions and behaviors toward everyone in our lives. Silently repeating compassionate phrases that convey our good wishes helps us to walk away from judging, resenting, or disliking, and move toward caring, connection, and understanding. Toward ourselves, toward others.

Raison is particularly interested in the benefits of loving-kindness meditation; his growing body of research indicates that developing this heightened sense of compassion toward others shifts our immune system in stunningly protective ways.

"Stress activates cytokine activity and inflammation, taxing your immune system in a way that's not all that different from what happens when you're infected by a virus or bacteria," Raison underscores the first time I speak to him by phone.

Let's say you cut your finger with a knife. Quickly, bacteria enter your body. Your immune cells, or macrophages, begin to secrete the inflammatory cytokines we're now familiar with, including IL-6 and IL-2. These cytokines and other chemicals flood the area in order to destroy the bacteria and stop their spread. But cytokines also damage the surrounding tissue, causing inflammation, which, unchecked, wreaks havoc on your body. This is why, Raison emphasizes, "Stress is implicated in every disease from depression to irritable bowel syndrome to autoimmune disease to heart disease to cancer."

Although mindfulness and meditation have long received a fair amount of attention from researchers, we have known less about the effects of compassion meditation on the mind and body.

Raison, who serves as the principal investigator in the largest federally funded study of compassion meditation, has set out to remedy that. He and his colleagues are working to quantify the effects of compassion meditation and the bidirectional relationship between stress and the depressive thought cycles that accompany stress, and the impact that stress hormones and other brain-produced chemicals have on the immune system and disease. Indeed, he may know more than anyone on the planet about how compassion meditation can change our brain and our cells and impact our health.

Raison recently took sixty-one healthy nineteen year-old students and gave half of them a six-week course in compassion meditation, while a control group took a health discussion course about health issues important to college students. Subjects in the compassion meditation group were asked to keep a diary of how often they practiced sending loving thoughts to themselves and others. At both the beginning and the end of the study, researchers gave participants a stress test, rating their psychological responses as they performed difficult math exercises and gave impromptu public speeches. At the end, researchers measured participants' blood levels of inflammatory chemical messengers, or cytokines, including interleukin IL-6, which, as we've seen, is higher when we're undergoing chronic stress.

Those who practiced compassion meditation for a total of an hour and a half to two hours over the course of each week "not only now saw stressful situations as less stressful, they also had lower levels of the inflammatory cytokine interleukin (IL-6), a chemical directly related to both inflammation and disease," Raison tells me.

Their PIN response went drastically down.

As with mindfulness and breath-based meditation, practicing compassion meditation allows us to react with greater equanimity and less negative emotion to difficult circumstances and challenging day-to-day interactions. Because we are actively sending thoughts of compassion to those around us, it may have the additional benefit of helping us to view the world in a more socially connected way, and to see the world around us as less threatening. "When you reinterpret the world as less dangerous, you don't get as much of a stress reaction," says Raison. By comparison, mindful breathing helps us to distance ourselves from negative or stressful thoughts. Each practice serves to take our disease-related stress hormone levels down to where they're no longer doing us mental and bodily harm.

In the process, we make room for joy and well-being.

"For most people the wear and tear of the modern world and our current lifestyles contribute significantly to disease," says Raison. He tells me, as an aside, that even the hours we spend commuting have been shown to contribute to much higher levels of inflammatory cytokines and stress hormones in our body. "The really great news is that we as human beings have evolved in such a way that we possess powerful tools in our human repertoire to shield ourselves against that wear and tear. Compassion meditation takes us back down to base, where we can deescalate that toxic, disease-promoting stress reactivity."

Raison, along with Geshe Lobsang Tenzin Negi, director of the Emory-Tibet Partnership, has been furthering research on loving-kindness meditation with a project called the Compassion and Attention Longitudinal Meditation Study, or CALM. Their current interest is investigating exactly which aspect of meditation is most responsible for the sorts of emotional, behavioral, and biological transformations that occur for those who practice. Actively sending compassion to the self and others that forms the bedrock of loving-kindness meditation? Or the practice of mindful breathing, which helps us to stop thoughts by focusing on the breath and center on the state of simply being? Or is it these practices in tandem that help us the most?

I THINK OF recent research on the power of the emotion of love on our body and brain. Stanford University Medical Center researchers

tell us that experiencing intense love provides startlingly effective relief from physical pain. Feelings of love for another activate the reward area of the brain in much the same way that painkillers—or
winning a lot of money—do.

It's certainly no surprise that stewing in hostile, angry feelings
hurts us. A study following nearly four thousand men and women for
ten years found that individuals who felt higher levels of anger and
hostility were more likely to develop heart problems.

Most of us can read that and reasonably reassure ourselves, *that's not
me.* But this same group of researchers found, more recently, that even
feeling higher levels of tension and anxiety predict a greater likelihood
of coronary heart disease, heart arrhythmia, and even death. And this
correlation between feeling anxious and a higher risk of mortality was
particularly true for women.

We fire up anxiety, tension, anger, and pain each time we dwell on
stressful thoughts, deepen the grooves in familiar, negative pathways
in the brain, and fill our bodies with inflammatory cytokines that do
damage to our bodies and may even shorten our telomeres.

Or we free ourselves from anxiety, tension, anger, and pain, and
quiet the brain, by calling forth compassion and love.

The brain on love, painkillers, or the lottery. Love is the only realistic option that doesn't come with side effects.

I DO NOT know how much the reading, investigating, and practicing
I've been doing plays into the life-changing decision that Zen and I
make the next day, but it factors in, somehow. I know it does.

For two years we've been toying with the idea of moving to Baltimore. I'm there every day—and it's where our kids go to school. It
might seem insane to allow your kids to ride a bus forty minutes each
way twice a day, but this school is that good—and the bus is full of
other kids doing the same. Still, the commute is wearing on them.

All of our living parents reside in Baltimore, and they are getting
older by the moment. Just recently, my mother was hospitalized for

high blood pressure and chest pains. My brothers are all an hour or two away.

My doctor appointments are all in Baltimore at Hopkins—including my many check-ins with Rowland-Seymour and all of my -ologists.

We have a joke that if I drive to Baltimore only once in a day that's a "onefer." Up and down twice in a day is a "twofer." Sometimes, I pull a "threefer." And that's pretty much a whole day in the car. It's hard on my body, my legs.

We've become a family of road warriors. The road time is killing us. I once added up all the hours that the kids spend on the bus, the hours I spend driving to school-related pickups, sports games, and evening events, doctor's appointments, and work and family visits in Baltimore—and among the three of us it came out to forty-five-plus hours a week.

Still, we're torn. Annapolis is home. I grew up on the Chesapeake Bay. I left for college and a publishing program that led to a decade of living and working in New York before I came home on a visit and met Zen by a fluke. It involved my puppy wrapping me up in the leash, my nearly falling over, Zen laughing, my untangling myself, and, ultimately, the dog falling asleep between Zen's feet as if to say, "home."

I stayed. Our friends from our past two decades—and from my growing up here—are precious to us. One of my brothers lives here, and our kids have been growing up together as only cousins can. That means everything.

Still, it's gotten to the point that we pretty much only sleep in Annapolis.

All this has been weighing on us. We've been making improvements around the house, just in case we find a house we like in Baltimore. But it's all been "What if?" rather than "We are."

Then today, out of the blue, we received an offer on our house from someone who heard we might be thinking of moving. Our house is not even on the market. It's not a great offer, but we're in the midst of the biggest housing slump in seventy-plus years so, as our Realtor—

and friend—who called to tell us about the offer reminds us, if we really do want to move . . . an offer is an offer.

Zen and I decide to take the leap of faith, jump off the cliff into the unknown—which is completely unlike us. Security and predictability are big pluses to us. Unlike many people in midlife we know how risky life can actually be. My dad died from routine surgery. When Christian was born he spent weeks in intensive care. I almost didn't get out of a wheelchair. My family lost all of its money overnight. Things go wrong. Life goes wrong.

But we need to carve out a life that takes place in two cities instead of three. As one of my friends puts it to me, "Your family lives in the car. And nothing really wonderful ever happened in a car, did it?"

We say yes to our Realtor.

"Is it normal to feel like you're going to throw up?" I ask her.

"Absolutely," she says.

I understand why they say moving is as stressful as having someone die—though having lived through both I would beg to differ. Of course it depends where you move—and who dies. Still, my heart is in my throat nearly every day at the idea of getting packed and out of here by our move date. It's a physical and emotional high jump.

Each time I look out over the kitchen sink, through the back window, I see our last golden retriever racing back and forth through the yard, chasing squirrels. I see the tea party I threw for Claire when she turned three, for which I made miniature cakes that looked like fine china teacups (in retrospect, perhaps as much for the sake of the other moms as for her). I see Christian and his friends collecting the loose branches in the yard and making a teepee that stayed up for a year. I see us blowing huge bubbles with a giant wand in full moonlight, Christian clapping each time one burst, calling out, "Mommy, the bubbles make the dark laugh!" The simple moments of a fairly cliché suburban life, I know. But it hurts to walk away from the setting of our best stories.

I am having a hard time moving on. How cliché I am.

And then I watch a chickadee I see from time to time hop from the hole it favors in our tree onto the deck rail and trill *chick-a-dee-dee-dee*.

It is trilling right here, right now. It seems to be trilling at me, *here you be-be-be*. Silly, I know. But it reminds me. I can use my awareness of what I'm feeling—*this is loss*—as one more blunt tool to beat myself up with, or I can marry my awareness to compassion. See myself with generosity. And instead of feeling stuck, move forward.

Move forward from the loss for a childhood that wasn't, the loss over my dad that lives forever, loss for my children's childhood, for the body I once had.

Moving on is going to be hard. Terrifying.

It seems like perfect timing when, in Trish's Friday morning class, we begin learning loving-kindness meditation—sending compassionate thoughts to ourselves, those we love, people we don't know well, and even to the folks who drive us absolutely nuts. The premise is that if we can tune into our innate desire to care for ourselves and to wish ourselves well, then we can, from there, connect with the inherent sense of worthiness within others despite their complex, human flaws.

In addition to classes, I've been practicing at an evening meditation group that Trish teaches, which, she has told us, is open to all her students as well as to everyone who meditates in the Baltimore community. This *sangha*—the Sanskrit word for a community that shares a common vision—practices both sitting and loving-kindness meditation together each week.

We begin by bringing our own image to mind and silently repeating each phrase to ourselves:

May I be filled with love and kindness.
May I be safe and protected.
May I love and be loved.
May I be happy and contented.
May I be healthy and strong.
May my life unfold with ease.

I repeat each sentiment, aware of a vague disconnect between what

I'm saying and what's sinking in. I feel guilty for not feeling more; for letting this be more recitation than meditation.

Then Trish asks us to add our own personal wish or blessing for ourselves. And really take it into our own heart.

May I be a person of joy. This is what comes to me. This is what I concentrate on. The desire floods me. *May I be a person of joy.*

I feel a warmth spreading through my body, the way you can feel certain meds spreading from an IV through your veins—only in this case it's a soft, welcome rush.

A realization hits me from nowhere, from underneath all the frenetic fear and thinking and ruminating and planning and fretting and anxious hum over moving and packing for the sake of my kids who spend too much time in the car and bus and don't deserve to spend their childhood caught in the juggernaut of the beltway. For my mother and in-laws who are all nearing eighty and who have no other children nearby and need someone in case of an emergency. *I must be a really good person. Because I really care about all these people.*

I am not sure when I last thought of myself as *a good person.*

Next, we focus our attention on someone for whom our love flows easily. Maybe not every moment of our lives but generally speaking. Someone we find it easy to send loving messages to. A child, a dear friend, even a pet.

This is so easy for me. I have only to think of my son, my daughter.

Safe and protected, healthy and strong—these have been something of our family leitmotif.

I think of the day we finally got to take Christian home from intensive care at Hopkins when he was seven weeks old. *Safe and protected.* I think of Claire's allergies and always keeping the EpiPen handy. *Healthy and strong.*

I think of the emotional bruises and paper cuts: the golden retrievers that died way too young from cancer, the childhood friends who moved away. Putting emotional bandages on each of these and promising them that tomorrow would be better. And it almost always was.

Happy and contented.

It's all inside them. It's all inside me.

I don't think these thoughts of well-being for my son, my daughter. I *am* these wishes. Like every mother on the planet these hopes for my children are woven into my cellular DNA.

Trish asks us to add our own silent, personal wish for the person we're sending love to. This, also, is easy for me.

May you each be a person of joy.

Because I am learning that everything else flows from that.

She asks us, next, to think of someone we barely know; someone we don't have strong positive or negative feelings toward. The school bus driver, the clerk in the post office, the UPS driver, the guy we see walking the dog in the neighborhood but have never met—or perhaps the person sitting next to us as we practice meditation.

I bring to mind the ever-helpful secretary at my children's school who is one of the kindest people I've ever met. She gives them messages for me, delivers forgotten items, and acts like a mom on an as-needed basis for hundreds of children. She has a saying, "We only have four years to love them." I smile, sending her these wishes of well-being without her even knowing. It feels as if I'm sending her an anonymous gift in the mail.

Finally, Trish asks us to move our attention to someone who is difficult in our lives. Someone with whom we feel friction, or even anger. It may be someone with whom we have a current argument or rift. "It's not necessary to pick the most difficult person in your life," she reassures us. "That may be too difficult. But someone who, if you stretch yourself, you feel you could send these well wishes to."

I am stymied for a minute. There have been troubling people in my life who, if I think about it, make me feel fairly crazy. But I don't see them much, or try not to, and so it's not so hard to put old wounds behind me.

The difficult thing for me is letting the more immediate crazy-making situations go. The client who bailed on a big project because he was, he said, having an emotional crisis. For a month he couldn't be found by either the publisher or me. Finally, the publisher gave up.

Which meant I didn't get paid for the months of work I'd done in good faith. When the client surfaced he was contrite, weepy, sorry, not at all well, and practically penniless he said—and I felt sorry for him. I comforted him over the phone. And then he flew off to give a speech that, a third party confided, paid him four times what he owed me. Later, I heard he was sailing in Fiji. Nothing like that had ever happened in my work life before. Working out the pity I felt for him (he was really not a well person, I knew that to be true) and the fact that I now had to face juggling our own household bills—all that, plus being lied to—now that's the kind of situation that makes me really, really crazy.

Suddenly, I feel sweaty and tense. My breath grows uneasy. My thoughts are revving up to 150 miles an hour. I start to replay the stupid excuses he's made. The way he played me, stupid me. It is a ludicrous waste of time, but nevertheless I rewind the tapes over and over in my mind. *How could he lie like that? How ridiculous! How dare he! Does he really think anyone believes a word he says? I did!* I am seething. And he's not even here in the room.

I think of the words of the Buddhist teacher Tsoknyi Rinpoche, the inheritor of one of the most distinguished family lineages in a long line of great Buddhist teachers.

He confesses in his teachings that even he knows what it's like to feel that something is so upsetting he can't let go. "There is this person," he says, in his strong, broken accent, "who vexes you. Lots of drama attached. Say it's 'John.'" It feels, in your body, he says, as if "John is driving a truck through you. *Vroom.* Every time you think of John you have this *vroom* feeling of a truck driving through you."

Vroom, vroom. That's it exactly. It's as if he's driving a Mac truck through my chest. *Vroom.*

"Try, if it's comfortable," Trish is saying in the meditation room, "to bring this person's image into your heart."

I don't want a lying Mac truck-driving liar in my heart. If he were standing in front of me right now I think I'd punch him!

May you be safe and protected.

May you be happy and contented.

May you be healthy and strong.

Trish asks us to add our personal wish for this person. *May you never contact me again.* Clearly I've failed; it's my fault for choosing someone who makes me so mad it's a stretch for me to send heartfelt well wishes to him in the first place, I suppose.

Forgiven.

I reassure myself with this thought: if the act of wishing a hurtful person in our lives well is part of the foundation of an ancient Buddhist practice thousands of years old, then we humans have been feeling like other people are driving a Mac truck (or a herd of buffalo) through our chests since the beginning of mankind. If what evolutionary biologists tell us is true—we evolved to have high threat reactivity in order to stay in the gene pool—then I am not alone, I am not that much more awful than any other ancient or modern human.

I remind myself, *he is not here. I am not my thoughts.* It is only the state of my mind, my anxiety, that's working me up until I feel as if I really have something to dread right here, right now. Just states of mind like any other. No more, no less. *They are not me.*

Trish asks us to bring our attention back to the center of our chest and imagine that our desire to wish others well is now expanding out beyond the boundaries of our body in all directions—to our left, right, in front of us, and in back of us.

I focus on her instructions. "Imagine that this is occurring effortlessly, just based on our intention to wish others well," she coaches. "And send these wishes now to all beings everywhere, without exception."

May all beings be filled with love and kindness.

I think of all the angry, lonely, suffering people everywhere who lack love, food, water, the basic right to live according to their free will. The direness of someone playing people with pity stories pales. The *vroom* dissipates.

All people, everywhere.

I am still aware of the person who drives through my chest, but my churning images of his face before my face slowly glide away. It's as if he has moved halfway across the room, rather than sitting here in front of me or, worse yet, inhabiting the inner walls of my mind. His image floats further off. And that's shocking. Because usually once I think of the entire situation, I can lose half an hour ruminating. But . . . suddenly . . . all thoughts of him . . . evaporate.

I feel a small trickle of compassion for him, being caught up in a habit of mind that comes from the ways in which he himself feels afraid and overly reactive and alone in his paper-tiger world and, as a result, lets himself and others down.

It is a relief to let go of the anger I've carried for weeks without even acknowledging it's infiltrated my being. My muscles, tendons, cells.

The antidote to anger is kindness.

I'm expanding. Beyond my own cell walls, wide, vast, free. I breathe out as I send well wishes to all beings. It feels surprisingly fluid to me. Natural. It feels necessary and good and . . . as if I'm giving oxygen to some vital part of *me.* For a moment, I lose all sense of space and time.

May all beings be safe and protected. I imagine the person who has caused me such angst in a light in the center of the circle of this consciousness, this space without walls. I know he has alienated colleagues, friends. I know he must feel very alone. *I feel so much compassion for him.*

And as I do I feel my heart reach out to the whole world—that larger, pulsing consciousness again—startling me, inviting me, drawing me. What is this place? What power is it that I feel is so intensely here?

And then the bell rings.

I have forgotten about the house, the move, the fear. I am thinking just about love.

Staying Out in Front of Myself

It's a good time to stop and appreciate what's working.

In the midst of utter chaos, the house was packed, the moving vans came and—we're temporarily living in a tiny townhouse while we wait for the county to approve our plans to build. That's right. Zen's parents have given us a small tract of land, parceled off of a much larger piece they own; it's five minutes from our kids' school, ten minutes from Hopkins, and near all three of our living parents. It's lovely of them to do this.

So. We are building a house. A modest house on a small piece of land. Getting closer to our school community, our family, spending less time on the road.

The bad news: we first have to develop the property. There are environmental protection issues to be mindful of regarding well, septic, forest buffer, storm-water management, soil erosion, and more. This could take us, we've just been told, a year—likely more. Camping out in a two-bedroom townhouse with most of our goods in storage while we sort this out is not ideal. I miss the trees, the yard, the birds. It reminds me of a saying I once heard: "You get out of one tight space only to squeeze into another one." A year plus is a long time.

Positivity time.

• • •

I've been reading the work of a researcher, Barbara Fredrickson, PhD, who has spent a decade in her lab studying the effects our positive emotions have on us. Fredrickson, whose research is funded by grants from the National Institute of Mental Health, takes a different track in showing the relationship between mindset and physical well-being. She believes that what matters most in terms of our well-being is our "positivity ratio."

Fredrickson uses this ratio as a way to judge the amount of an individual's "heartfelt positivity" relative to the amount of his or her "heart-wrenching negativity." Stated formally, she explains, our positivity ratio is our frequency of positive thoughts over any given time span, divided by our frequency of negative thoughts over that same time span. Or P over N (mathematically, P/N).

Fredrickson has found, after studying hundreds of people each year, that the P/N that leads to overall positivity is three to one. When we have three times more positive thoughts than negative, we "take off, drawn along an upward spiral energized by positivity," she says. Our behavior and problem-solving skills not only become more creative, we feel more uplifted, more alive.

When our P/N quotient plunges below this ratio, we hit a tipping point. Our overall life view skews toward the negative. We get pulled into a downward spiral that becomes fueled by more negativity. So much so that our response and behavior become, she says, "painfully predictable." We feel burdened. We can't make good choices. Our creative juices and sense of humor dry up. We feel . . . lifeless.

That downward spiral becomes more and more difficult to stop as it picks up momentum.

Beyond the pleasant feeling we get when we tune into positivity, the process has a powerful physical effect. Even mild and fleeting moments of positivity are more potent than we know and are one more way to usher in a positive floating brain, and move away from a negative PIN response.

A recent review of research on how positive emotions influence health outcomes found that people with stronger positive emotions have lower levels of chemicals associated with inflammation related to stress. Some studies suggest positive emotions even undo some of the physical damage and inflammation previously caused by stress.

Being grateful for and acknowledging what's positive in your life is likewise nourishing. People who make it a habit to express gratitude are happier, healthier, and better able to withstand life's downturns.

Negativity, on the other hand, borrows from our future. It's another tool in the joy thief's hands.

Perhaps the most prolific researcher who has worked to show the link between positivity and well-being is Martin Seligman, psychologist and director of the Positive Psychology Center at the University of Pennsylvania. In the mid-1980s, Seligman and his then graduate student at Penn, Gregory Buchanan, were interested in a previously done study on a group of 120 men from San Francisco who had suffered their first heart attacks. These men had been interviewed on videotape about their families, jobs, and hobbies. Seligman and Buchanan looked at each patient's videotape and coded statements for optimism or pessimism. They then sealed up their coded reports and put them away.

Eight and a half years passed before they opened the files again. By then, half of the men had died from a second heart attack. Seligman wanted to know, could they predict who would have a second heart attack? It turned out that the usual risk factors—blood pressure, cholesterol, how serious the first heart attack had been—did not predict the likelihood of a second heart attack. The single most significant predictor of who would face a second cardiac event was optimism. Of the sixteen most pessimistic men, fifteen died. Of the sixteen most optimistic men, only five died. In another cardiovascular disease study, which tracked over thirteen hundred veterans for ten years, men with the most optimism had 25 percent fewer episodes of cardiovascular disease.

The reasons behind these robust findings for optimism and health, says Seligman, are threefold. First, optimists believe that their actions matter, whereas pessimists tend to lapse into what Seligman calls "passive helplessness." This means optimists are more likely to act on medical advice, give up smoking, take better care of themselves, diet, exercise regularly, and protect sleep habits—all of which lead to better health outcomes.

Second, optimists tend to have more social support. The more friends you have in your life, the healthier you tend to be. Not surprising, given what we have learned from our investigations into loving-kindness and compassion meditation, the more love in our life, the less illness. As one famous study by Harvard psychologist George Vaillant shows, having just one person in your life whom you feel comfy calling at three a.m. to share a problem with correlates to better physical health.

And finally, of course, there is our immune function. Pessimists suffer more distress and stress. These repeated episodes of stress, particularly if one feels hopeless to change things, generate more stress hormones and inflammatory cytokines such as IL-6 and IL-2, leading to long-lasting inflammation and disease. Indeed, inflammation is directly implicated in atherosclerosis. And women who are more depressed and feel like they don't have control over their lives have greater signs of calcification damage in the major arteries of their hearts.

RESEARCHERS HAVE SHOWN that positive mood also enhances creative problem solving and generates more "flexible yet creative thinking." Investigators recently elicited different mood responses from students by either showing them music clips that made them feel happy (a peppy Mozart piece, videos of laughing babies) or sad (music from *Schindler's List*, a news report about a devastating earthquake), or by showing them neutral music and videos that didn't make an impact on mood. After listening and watching, students had to try to learn to recognize a particularly difficult pattern.

Those who had been exposed to happy music and videos performed better when learning how to classify patterns than did sad or neutral volunteers because, researchers say, a happy mood helps us to think more innovatively. Which may be, they point out with all seriousness, why people tend to like to watch funny videos at work; they're unconsciously trying to put themselves in a good mood. (That means that when people cluster around someone's desk watching clips from *The Office* they're actually increasing their productivity, creativity, and problem-solving skills.)

Kindness to self, mindfulness and meditation, and loving-kindness are all impacting how I view the world. And myself. But I still wouldn't say I'm, in a word, positive. Or grateful. My positivity versus negativity ratio—my *P/N*—is certainly shy of the three positive outlooks on what's happening in my world to every one time I view things negatively.

I GET OUT a pad of sticky notes and put another yellow sticky on my steering wheel: *What's going right today?*

Today, I can answer:

One. I'm getting organized!

This goes beyond having gone through every file, dish, knick-knack, drawer, closet, cabinet, and item of clothing in our house and culling down to only what we need to live in a sixteen-hundred-square-foot apartment. Though I am proud of having successfully executed what I call the "house colonic."

I mean the organization of *me.* I am making real efforts to sit down and focus on the breath. Take mindful sighs. Catch my thoughts in midair. That's progress. Still, just as many days my plan to "sit later today" doesn't pan out very well. Fires are put out with a little mindfulness here, a little breathing there, while sparks of worry, fatigue, and fretting smolder and flame.

Two. I'm finding creative ways to work meditation in even when I can't "sit." When I walk the dogs (yes, dogs; we've acquired another rescue dog, a little sheltie and terrier mix named Winnie), I head to a scant patch of greenery near the townhouse we're renting. A small cluster of trees and bushes sits inside a square of sidewalk that's twenty feet long on each side. The tiny square is surrounded by a parking lot. I circle the minuscule garden, keeping my eyes softly focused. I move mindfully, practicing what Buddhists call walking meditation: to be conscious of how we move, the lifting of each leg, the arc of heel and toe, marrying it to our breath, feeling our body touch the earth, and touch it again. And as I go, I repeat the familiar phrases of compassion meditation. I realize it's all too like me to be doing three things at once: walking meditation, exercising dogs, practicing loving-kindness. Since I have multitasked my way through life for so long, it may be that my brain can no longer unitask.

And so I multimeditate.

I emerge from my multimeditation square a different person. My shoulders fall. My breath deepens. I feel myself taking a detour off the mental distress highway.

I am, perhaps, the crazy new lady in the neighborhood who walks in circles in the parking lot mumbling to herself. But it hardly matters. If someone stares at me wide-eyed from his or her car while driving past, I just send them stealth loving-kindness and my self-consciousness melts. *The antidote is compassion.*

It may not be textbook perfect, but multimeditating counts for progress. Trish, to whom I have confessed my multimeditating practice, tells me that combining walking and loving-kindness is a well-established, accepted form of meditation. There exists, in fact, a tradition of practicing compassion meditation throughout one's entire day, no matter what we're doing. Including walking the dogs.

Three. When I do "sit" I give myself the gift of going to the green. There are little park benches in my patch of green. When I sit and listen to the birds, the gentle music of the rustling trees, I meditate more deeply while nature nurtures.

Our cellular responses to being near nature are very different from those we have in urban settings. In Japan, physicians often prescribe twenty minutes of *shinrin-yoku*, or "forest bathing," for patients. It makes sense. Walking through a forest pumps up our parasympathetic nervous system and suppresses the sympathetic nervous stress-now system for hours and even days. We even do better on memory and attention tests after walking through natural settings. That's why when many of our first hospitals were built they included a sunroom or "solarium" where patients could view nature. Now we know those instincts were spot-on. Patients with a view of nature and trees heal more quickly, spend less time in the hospital, need fewer painkillers, and have fewer post-op complications than those who look out on an urban setting. When we seek out what researchers call "nearby nature"—which is usually free and accessible to most of us somewhere, somehow—we tend to be healthier overall and feel greater life contentment and satisfaction.

Four. Errands and human interactions are a lot more fun.

It's fun to see or talk to people right after you've sent them stealth loving-kindness. The clerk at the dry cleaner who is usually surly to every customer suddenly seems to be smiling. The writing client who is usually so unpleasant it makes editors cringe cracks a joke in a meeting. The unhappy person behind me in line at the grocery store who spends five minutes grumbling because I have nine items instead of eight in my cart and am in the under-eight-items line (I confess, I neglected to count the magazine with the cover story on dog rescue that Claire threw in at the last minute) suddenly smiles and shrugs for me to go ahead. Once I've sent someone an anonymous dose of loving-kindness, it changes me and alters what happens the next time we interact.

Similarly, running errands has gone from being an almost unbearable time suck to an opportunity to connect, to see how others change me and my way of being in the world, and how my small, intentional kindnesses change them. A smile, a door opened, a "Have a great day!" A moment taken to pick up a stuffed animal for a toddler who dropped it from a shopping cart, or sharing my umbrella, yesterday, with a stranger while we waited to run from the grocery store to our cars. Errands are an opportunity to spread a layer of kindness over what sometimes seems a grim, tense, honking, and unhappy world.

There is a Buddhist saying that "When I awakened the whole world awakened with me." It's as if we're all just waiting for everyone else to smile first.

That makes me think of a line from an Alice LaPlante novel: "I am a visitor from another planet, and the natives are not friendly." Sometimes we all feel this way. But the question is, Are we friendly? Am I?

Five. Moments of thinking, *I love my life*.

It will happen at the oddest times. I watch Zen, Christian, and Claire load food into the car for Thanksgiving dinner at my brother's. I see how beautiful they are, how they work in tandem as a family does, their arms transferring boxes one to the other, arranging them in the seats, loading up the dogs, the smell of still-steaming pumpkin pie rising in the cold air. Claire raises her nostrils to take in the smell: "Pie!" she exclaims to the universe, arms flung out. There is a reason we call Claire our family joystick. She has a way of revving good moments into great ones.

The thought *I love my life* flashes through my brain.

This is no small thing. Because I often catch myself starting a thought with the words "I hate. . . ." *I hate that, I hate it when, I hate how.*

I love my life lasts for only a minute or two. As I lift the two bags of salad makings and extra dinner dishes I'm carrying, a wave of fatigue whooshes through me, nearly buckling my legs. The tendonitis in my wrists screams. I set down the bags before I drop my best china on the driveway and fake a smile, putting a good face over a tired body, until the bottom-dropping-out feeling wanes; I don't want anyone to see my eyes gray. Other frettings set in. I realize we are running late (again), and I forgot the salad dressing (again). An argument breaks out in the backseat. I look down at my black pants and dark-gray sweater, magnets for dog hair, wishing that my closet had magically produced something I wanted to wear—though of course that would mean actually going shopping. I look in the car mirror and see that the rash on my face is so terrible I'm not sure what people will think or if they will even want to shake my hand. But the fact is that for one small instant the feeling *I love my life* was there.

Six. I am hugging my family a lot. This starts Zen joking, "I need more vitamin D" (D, as in Donna). This expands into a larger family joke that we both need more vitamin C (yes, Christian and Claire).

When we call for a group family hug, Christian and Claire both pretend to protest. Claire's head falls against her brother's chest. They share a small, knowing sigh. *The things our parents make us do.* Wrapping my arms around them, even though Christian is six feet tall, still growing, and more than halfway through high school, is a little like trying to hold the whole dancing-away world in my arms.

Zen's instincts are right. Hugs are vitamins. Especially long hugs. I've read that the average hug lasts three seconds, but longer hugs—twenty seconds—do us the most good. They increase levels of the bonding hormone oxytocin, which in turn lowers our levels of cortisol. Just a soft touch sends a shot of oxytocin into our bloodstream that's so powerful that people playing investment strategy games are more willing to hand over their money to strangers. Women who get more hugs from their husbands have higher levels of oxytocin, lower blood pressure, and less risk of heart disease— benefiting from hugs even more than men do. I'll take all the vitamin C—and Z—I can get.

Seven. I have an emergency toolbox.

When I feel myself becoming overwhelmed I draw upon my newly developed emergency mental repair plan. I do best when I use several of my favorite tricks in sequence to switch my brain from SNS/negative floating brain/Pain Channel to PNS/positive floating brain/Life Channel. It goes something like this:

1. Let out three rapid-fire exhales in the Tibetan Buddhist tradition. Or, three mindful sighs.
2. Rock a little, just for a minute or two. I haven't read this anywhere; I just came to this one day on my own. A slight back and forth, back and forth. I can't hold a grudge or fear when I'm rocking. Maybe that's why we rock children in our lap, or why we like to rock on the porch when we are old. Rocking calms us. Our fears let go their tentacle hold.
3. Roll my eyes just slightly up toward the top of my head as I'm focusing on the breath. I've stumbled across this by trial and

error as well. When I do a little research on why this brings on a sudden wave of calm, what I read makes sense. Rolling our eyes slightly upward triggers relaxation—that's why when we sleep our eyes roll up toward the top of our head.

4. Touch my fingers to my lips, gently, as I might if I were saying *shhhhhhhhh* to a small, distressed child. Touching our lips stimulates the parasympathetic nerve fibers that line them. That's why babies love to self-soothe by breast-feeding, and suckling on their fingers and pacifiers.

5. Imagine a golden white column of light streaming into my scalp and crown—traveling all the way down through my chest into my belly, touching every cell of my body, moving into my toes, and finally shooting down into the ground.

6. If I am not outside, I imagine myself in nature.

7. If I am very sad, I imagine the faces of the people who have really, really loved me. Surrounding me. Wishing the best for me.

8. Focus on the sounds that surround me, whether real or in my imagined scenery.

9. Use word power. Name my habits of mind. Apply balm to the sting.

10. Come back to the breath. *This in breath, this out breath.*

11. If necessary, begin at the top and work my way down again.

Eight. "You yell a lot less than you used to."

Driving to school, Christian tells me, out of the blue, "I notice you yell a lot less than you used to."

"Yeah," Claire pipes in from the backseat, agreeing, on this rare occasion, with her brother. "You don't sound so much like Charlie Brown's teacher. *WaaWaaWaaWaaWaa*." I glance at her in the rearview mirror. Her mouth is moving like a fish blowing air bubbles.

I think back to a scene a few days earlier. I am standing in the kitchen emptying the dishwasher when Christian, who is flipping through the *New Yorker*, absentmindedly picks up one of Claire's EpiPens, and says, "Oh, is this a practice Epi?"

Claire has an anaphylactic allergy to peanuts and hazelnuts. EpiPens save her life because they're preloaded with epinephrine, or adrenaline, the same hormone our body produces when we enter fight or flight. Only the Epi delivers a large dose very quickly, in a shorter time than our body can. The injection dampens the allergic and immunologic response, preventing the throat from closing up. The heart begins to race and blood floods into the muscles. Once administered, the patient feels fluttery and agitated—and needs to get to an emergency room because the effects of all that pumped-up stress hormone have to be closely monitored.

"No!" I shout as my son jabs the EpiPen toward the palm of his hand. I take a leap toward him over the dishwasher door that lies open between us.

"Mom!" he cries as the EpiPen goes off.

"Christian!" I trip toward him, grabbing his palm, trying to find where the needle has penetrated. The cover of the *New Yorker* grows dark and wet as the Epi's contents soak across it. My heart is racing. The needle, having just missed his palm, is protruding from the caricature of a large turkey gracing the magazine's Thanksgiving week cover. "What were you *thinking*?!"

"Mom, I'm sorry!"

"*Christian!*" I am shouting.

"I'm really sorry, Mom. That was so *stupid*."

That was so stupid. I stop. I glance up at him. I watch—as if in slow motion—as his jaw grows long, and the wince of self-recrimination clouds his eyes.

I have a flash recollection of a line in writer Anne Lamott's book, *Imperfect Birds*. A teen deep in the awkward, heavy feelings of adolescent not-okay-ness asks an adult she trusts what "the secret" is. To living. Her grown-up friend whispers simply three words to her: "You are preapproved."

You are preapproved. I don't believe I have sent this message. Or at least not enough. I think I have been a mindless fit-to-be-tied mom more than I should.

"I thought it was a practice Epi . . . I wanted to try using it in case I ever have to help Claire," he blurts out.

I turn to face him. I give him the longest hug. He is so tall now he has to lean down in a lumbering sort of way to rest his head on my shoulder, but he manages it all the same. "Listen to me," I say, holding my strapping boy to me. "Number one. I'm sorry I yelled."

"Number two. In the future, never pick up a medical device without asking first. No exceptions."

He nods. "Good idea." He stands straighter to look at me, though only one side of his lips smile, like an apostrophe.

"Third, remember this: sometimes, very occasionally, we all act without thinking. We make mistakes in what we say, what we think, what we do, how we react. We all have our fifteen-year-old moments. Even when we're fifty."

He looks at me, considering. "Okay," he says. His eyes slide off in that sideways teenager gaze that says, *Is this going to be one of those awkward parent-advice talks?*

"Last and most important thing. You are preapproved." I pause. "Just as you are."

He starts to do an eye roll that's not an eye roll because eye rolling isn't allowed. It's what I call, instead, the "stroll"—half eye roll, half side stare.

"You are *preapproved*."

This time he looks me in the eye. Searching for something.

"As for the rest, it's all just a learning experience," I say. "But usually, it's better to practice on oranges."

Both sides of his mouth smile. We both burst out laughing.

You yell a lot less than you used to.

IF I AM now a mom who yells less than she used to, then I am getting closer to whom I want to be.

And that must mean my cells are getting closer to what I hope they'll become, too.

· 14 ·

The Black Ferret

"The amazing thing," Anastasia Rowland-Seymour is saying, in between listening to my chest inhalations with her stethoscope, "is that you are doing as well as you are."

Every three months or so I loop back to her for a checkup, in addition to regular e-mail check-ins. She's concerned about the impact the move has had on me, physically and emotionally.

I've told her that I sorted through eleven years of stuff and packed for nine hours a day for six weeks. My mother, nearly eighty years old, packed up the dining room dishes—most of which were hers or my grandmother's. Zen and my brothers hauled things to Goodwill. The kids boxed up old toys for charities. But mostly I packed it all, closet by closet, room by room.

And the thing is, I did not collapse. Many times over the past few months I went up and down the stairs without having to lie down at the top.

"Six months ago—even three months ago—could you have done all this?" Rowland-Seymour asks, wrapping her stethoscope around her shoulders.

I consider this. "Not without a major flare-up, no. I don't think I could have." I have had several friends tell me the same: *I was so afraid you would end up back in the hospital.*

"I feel better physically. I can do more. I'm not lying down every day." I stop for a moment to think about it. I'm having far fewer "maybe" and "I'm-not-sure-yet-if-I-can-do-that" days. "That's enormous," I explain, "and a gift I didn't expect."

"What strategies do you find are helping you the most?"

I think about it for a moment. "Everything is helping, bit by bit. But certain things stand out for me as quick-release strategies—tools I can count on to shift my state of mind and my energy level when everything seems too much," I say.

"Walking meditation tops the list," I start. "Let's say it's time to serve dinner and I haven't gotten half of what I needed to do done for work so I'm cranky, and the contractor calls to say, 'Oh, bad news, the electric company won't hook us up for another month so all interior work is stalled'—*ka-ching!*—and Zen is grumpy because it's already eight o'clock at night and no one has eaten, and I am mad because he could have moved dinner along faster if he'd just put down his guitar and noticed how much I had going on, and Christian needs to be picked up in twenty minutes from play practice, and that flu-like exhaustion from having been on my legs without stopping since seven a.m. is rising like a wave . . ."

Rowland-Seymour gives a little knowing laugh.

"The answer used to be lying down." I pause, taking in a deep breath after my unloading. "But now it's walking meditation.

"Because I can really do it. I can fit it in, and the dogs always need a walk, even if someone else has to stir the chili while I head out." I know that concentrating on the feel of my feet touching the pavement and sending thoughts of loving-kindness is going to take my PIN response right down. And when I take it down I feel more energetic. And when I feel more emotionally and physically energetic I can handle everything that's coming at me with more grace and good will.

She is still smiling. I am not the same woman she met six months ago. That woman would never have left the chili for someone else to stir.

"And going to my *sangha*," I continue. That surprises me, a little, I confess. "I don't know the people well, except for Trish, and a few compatriots from my MBSR class who I feel a certain connection to, but it's not a time for sharing or friendship. It's about being in the same safe space with people of like mind, searching for the same peace together. I feel better just entering the door."

"Can you set up a regular meditation space at home, so that whenever you sit there, you tap into that sense that you are here for that one purpose, which, in turn, will start to have that same portal effect?"

I agree, having a distinct meditation space set up at home—other than Zen's and my bed, which, I confess, is usually taken over by people studying for tests or reading books or playing board games—would help. But, I tell her, "in our crunched living space that is not going to happen. Not until we move. My favorite meditation space is a bench outside."

"So, go to your bench more," she says. She gives a tap with a small, silver reflex hammer on each of my knees. My lower-leg reflexes are often iffy. "Very good!" she says, as each lower leg flies out, first one, then, tap, the other. "Very nice!"

"And when you can't go outside?" she asks. "Or it's not a *sangha* night?"

"You mean when I'm driving or stuck in line or have to be somewhere in two minutes?"

"Exactly."

"Watching my thoughts. Relabeling. Taking in a deep breath. Staying with it. If I can't stay with it, bringing in a breath exercise," I say. "If one doesn't work, the combination of all the breath exercises I know always works—and, assuming I keep my eyes open, it's a good way to pass the time while driving." I feel a little lift, having relayed how much I've learned, appreciating how much it's really working for me. "But still . . ." There is, in my good report, something I'm not saying.

"But?" she asks when I fall quiet.

"Well, for all the gains I've made in terms of not feeling as fatigued and flu-ish, I have moments when I feel more . . . blue-ish." I am thinking of the deep layer of sadness that sometimes creeps up. That terrible, heavy feeling. Like some *thing* is inside. That black ferret, stretching, pawing, awakening in my brain. As if it's trapped there. And it can't get out.

She continues her checkup as we talk. Her fingers are warm and gentle as she reaches down to take my pulse.

"For a long time I've lived on what I think of as the Pain Channel," I tell her. "Now that it isn't blaring quite as loudly, I'm seeing that something else is there. Something quieter, deeper."

"Something that maybe the pain and illness have been covering up?" she asks.

"I'm not sure." I tell her about the word *forgiven*, how it makes my body ache, tears leak. "I thought that mindfulness and meditation would open me up to joy, lighten my load," I try to jest, but my voice catches. "In so many moments I do feel more alive, calmer, less anxious. But what I didn't anticipate was . . . more sadness. The antithesis to joy."

She is quiet as she tilts my head up to get a better look at the rash that snakes down my face and below my chin. The peeling puffer fish chin, the red scaly eyes, the red rash below my nose that makes it seem as if I have a permanent cold. I've shown her the three most recent creams I've bought to help battle my eczema so I won't wake up clawing my skin at night. The small, earnest Indian woman in the health-food store where I sometimes shop told me that with these she'd had "one-hundred-percent success with eczema." So I spent sixty dollars. But they haven't worked. Nothing has.

Rowland-Seymour signals for me to get down from the exam table. I settle myself in the chair next to her desk.

"You've spent the last few months focusing so intently on organizational details, from moving your family to the plans for building a house," she says. "Your practices are working, but they're worked in around everything else, and that doesn't allow a lot of time for reflection. Right now, you need to focus an equal amount of intensity on going inside, on being introspective with yourself. When you do, you may find some layer you haven't yet uncovered." She pauses. I sense she wants to say more.

"My skin is a barometer for something deeper that hasn't yet healed?"

Her palms turn a smidge upward as if to say she can't be certain. "It's a protective barrier that won't mend. You may need to take a detour on your journey to find out what's beneath that wounded layer, what keeps erupting, and why."

"Do I have time for all that?" I have only one year. I am about to incorporate yoga and acupuncture. There is a lot left to investigate.

"I don't think you have time *not* to," she says. "Otherwise whatever keeps coming up will keep getting in your way. You may have to deal with the pain to get closer to the joy. Otherwise it may be that nothing you try will ever really stick."

I have wondered since we first met if Rowland-Seymour's interest in the newly understood link between childhood adversity and adult illness might be born as much from personal experience as keeping abreast with the current literature.

"You've had to figure that out for yourself?" I ask.

"I've lost both parents." She pauses. "They each struggled with their own mental health challenges. It's hard to make sense of what's happening when you're very young." For a moment there is a liquid quality in her brown eyes that I haven't seen before. It clicks into place then: why she seemed so quick to understand when I first sketched out the details of my own childhood to her. Why she's taken on this quest with me. She's been in that childhood, too. She has her own details.

"I'm so very sorry." I know from having been on the receiving end all my life that there are no right words. But there is, it comes to me, right thinking: *May you be surrounded by love and kindness. May you be at ease.*

"Seeing what's beneath the sadness that keeps coming up may be one of the most important steps you take," she says, getting back to the matter at hand. "Whatever is there has probably been there all along. Have you seen Marla Sanzone yet?"

When we first began this quest, Rowland-Seymour and I agreed I would visit with Marla Sanzone, PhD, a psychotherapist who often works with patients who've experienced physical illness, helping them to grasp the relationships among childhood history, chronic illness, and mood. I worked with Sanzone several years ago, when I was still actively recovering from the paralysis of Guillain-Barré. She helped me find the courage and wisdom to respond to Zen's, Christian's, and Claire's grief and fear at the same time that I was collapsing under my own.

Yes, I had followed up on Rowland-Seymour's suggestion to see Dr. Sanzone. We met several weeks ago to establish a "joy index"—an inventory to determine the prevalence of my positive feelings of joy, contentment, and well-being, as well as my negative feelings of sadness and anxiety. We have another meeting scheduled next week to go over her findings. Then, at the end of my year, I'll retake the joy inventory and Sanzone will compare my before and after scores, to see if and how my worldview has changed.

Rowland-Seymour and I talk about the recent research on the power of words, and how the more we utilize the area of our brain that verbally names our feelings, the freer we are from the emotions themselves; the less they rule our state of mind and our life. A great deal of recent research has looked at the power of naming what we feel in relationship to mindfulness and meditation. Meanwhile, analogous work has been going on in the field of talk therapy as well, with equally robust findings.

We decide that I will:

1. Set up several talk therapy sessions with Sanzone.
2. Spend more time in private reflection and try dropping in the questions: What's going on inside? What am I feeling, and what is this feeling really about? Trish hinted when we first began to

work together months ago that if difficult emotions did start to arise as my meditation practice grew, I'd be more resilient and able to deal with them because I'd have the necessary tools. Do I have those tools yet? And how will I know?

Rowland-Seymour suggests that I might benefit from a short meditation retreat, and I recall that there is a women's winter meditation retreat coming up with psychologist and meditation teacher Tara Brach—the author of *Radical Acceptance*, which I read at Trish's suggestion. I brighten at the idea. I loved reading her book and speaking with her afterward. Tara is, I've been told by members of my *sangha*, well-known for asking retreat students to drop in tough questions during their meditations in order to break through to a deeper level of self-awareness. Rowland-Seymour likes the idea of my having forty-eight hours away from my family to see what might emerge when I'm not triaging family matters. We both know that's as much time as I can take away given work, family, and financial constraints. The fee is reasonable, and we agree I'll sign up. I confess to her that this will be my first time away from my family in fifteen years—except for trips to the hospital or to lecture.

3. Yoga, yoga, yoga. It's time to get my wobbly legs on the mat, and see what comes of that.
4. I'll also begin weekly acupuncture. There is a great deal of science on the benefits of acupuncture. Here, too, we know where to start. Janet Althen, MAc, LAc, Dipl. Ac., founder of a women-only acupuncture clinic, practices not far from where I now live. She's a local legend for the photo array of newborn babies in her office—pictures given to her by moms who'd been battling infertility for years when they first came for treatment. She's also known for helping women with fatigue, thyroiditis, arthritis—and hot flashes.

· 15 ·

More Than Skin Deep

I'm curious about why Rowland-Seymour kept hinting at a relationship between my skin and mood, and even decade-old emotions.

I think of the idioms referring to the mind-skin relationship that float through our cultural lexicon. "He gets under my skin." "I'm itching to do it." "It makes my skin crawl just to think of it." So often the premises behind our old, familiar adages turn out to be supported by today's new brain research, proving that our human instincts are eerily on target.

Such is the case with the relationship between skin and the brain—indeed, neuroscientists have isolated such profound relationships among skin, mood, and emotion that many have begun to refer to the skin as the "brain on the outside."

In the past decade researchers have come to understand that the skin is a source and target of neurotransmitters and neurohormones that were previously thought to be the domain of the central nervous system. When changes take place in our brain, changes take place in our skin. When we feel psychological stress, our brain reacts by sending signals directly to our skin so that it will respond as if we're under physical attack. That's why we flush red when we're embarrassed or angry or weepy. When we're afraid, color drains from our face. A teenager's skin breaks out before finals or the prom. Psychological stress worsens symptoms of skin disorders such as psoriasis and eczema.

Whenever we're under stress and the negative floating brain gets activated, the brain's amygdala increases production of a protein called neuropsin. This protein triggers a series of chemical events that turn on genes that determine the stress response on a cellular level throughout our body. When researchers look at normal skin, they find weak levels of neuropsin. However, the expression pattern of neuropsin is significantly higher in skin afflicted with chronic skin conditions including psoriasis, seborrheic keratosis, and the autoimmune disease lichen planus.

It strikes me as apropos that this amygdala-driven cellular response would afflict our skin in profound ways: the skin constitutes 6 percent of our total body weight and is the largest organ of the body. It contains a lot of our cells.

Psychiatrist Daniel Amen, MD, author of over a dozen studies examining how our brain activity changes with state of mind, and the author of the popular book *Change Your Brain, Change Your Life*, tells the story of a U.S. Army colonel he once treated at the Walter Reed Army Medical Center who had a rash all over his body that wouldn't resolve despite every known treatment. His wife had died a few years earlier in a car accident, and Amen came to discover that he had never cried or allowed himself to grieve over her death. He'd been left a widower with four children to raise. He had a quite demanding job that required his full attention. His conscious mind simply would not allow him to face his emotions out of fear that if he did, he would lose total control of his life. Eventually, through the use of hypnosis therapy, which bypassed his conscious need to maintain utter control over his environment, Amen was able to help the colonel grieve for the first time. He spent five therapy sessions simply sobbing, feeling the loss of his best friend and spouse. Over the next several months of letting his grief surface, his rash disappeared.

Other significant studies on a brain-skin link have been done in

Sweden, where researchers have been able to diagnose bipolar disorder by looking at specific skin cells rather than taking tissue samples from brain matter. Certain skin cells mirror brain cells, functioning similarly to the brain cells that are believed to be involved in bipolar disorder and schizophrenia. That's because our skin produces many of the same neuropeptides, such as melatonin and serotonin, that are produced by the brain.

I put in a call to Chuck Raison at Emory and ask him what he knows about the link between state of mind and emotion, and the skin. He tells me that some other very interesting work on skin and mood is being done by Christopher Lowry, PhD, in the Department of Integrative Physiology at the University of Colorado Boulder.

Lowry's work focuses on the relationships among serotonin levels in the brain, skin temperature, and depression. His recent paper, which has the entertaining title "That Warm Fuzzy Feeling: Brain Serotonergic Neurons and the Regulation of Emotion," shows a direct relationship between skin temperature and depression. Exposure to warm temperatures increases the activity of serotonin in a section of the brain known as the dorsal raphe nucleus, an area that Lowry suspects is related to depression. He believes that when this temperature-sensitive set of serotonin-producing neurons is dysregulated, we are more likely to experience anxiety and depression.

These findings make sense, he says, when we consider that people who are depressed often experience altered temperature cycles. Almost all antidepressants can cause a side effect of sweating, which happens when a thermoregulatory cooling mechanism is triggered in response to a signal that we are warm.

Lowry's work interests me deeply on a personal level. My skin is always cold. I am always cold. I wear sweaters even in the summer and each August Zen gives me another hand-knit cardigan because he knows I can never have enough. People often touch my hands and shrink back: *Whoa! Your hands are so cold!* I have heard this hundreds of times. Much of this is due to the two neurological diseases I've faced—small-fiber sensory neuropathy and Guillain-Barré. Both alter the nerve connections that help to conduct heat. For months after my second episode with GBS, my legs were blue and shockingly cold to the touch from the knee down.

I think of another word link. We refer to our skin as being blue when we are cold, and we call someone blue when he or she feels sad. Once again, our conversational expressions long precede the scientific discoveries that later support them—showing us how prescient our human understanding is of the connections among mood, emotion, and physical well-being.

Daniel Amen has also written that your skin can likewise affect your brain. MRIs show that when we scratch our skin, we activate areas of the brain including the prefrontal cortex, inferior parietal lobe, and cerebellum.

What's most interesting about this latter fact, though, is that scratching also deactivates the anterior and posterior cingulate cortices, areas associated with unpleasant emotions and memories. Which means scratching can help us to keep unpleasant memories or sensations related to past trauma at bay.

This stops me.

I scratch all the time. *Scratch, scratch, scratch.*

Once I start thinking of skin-related analogies I can't stop. I recall how, when I was packing boxes for the move, I found old college term papers, teacher letters, letters from friends. I was stunned by the amount of anxiety that emerged from the pages of my old journals— over a job or a boss or a guy. The angst. But here's what really threw me: I found letters from professors who so believed in me, and though I remember each of them and their impact on me well, I don't remember ever absorbing the words I now see they took so much trouble to put on the page, their faith in who I was and what I might do. Worse, I found long letters from people I couldn't even remember knowing. The truth is, though I appeared to be a normal college girl, I was an anxious college girl still recovering from an anxiety-producing ACE-ripe childhood.

I wasn't in my own skin.

• • •

I RECALL READING the work of researchers at Cornell University, who recently discovered that during adolescence the brain actually employs mechanisms to suppress its most fearful memories and feelings. The brain literally blunts the synaptic activity in the amygdala, the fear center, dampening molecular signaling in the hippocampus, the brain region involved in retrieving fearful memories. Previously formed, traumatic emotional memories are pushed underground.

Think of it: our young brains sublimate the feelings that surround any early traumatic event so that we can get through the emotionally vulnerable coming-of-age years alive, grow up, and survive. Move into adulthood without, hopefully, throwing ourselves over the side of a bridge and removing ourselves from the gene pool.

Researchers say that our brain's ability to black out our darkest recollections reveals a "unique form of brain plasticity" during the adolescent years.

Meanwhile, there is an analogous tenet from the field of psychology that holds that when we are young and experience trauma, the stressful emotions that accompany those memories become embedded deep in our bodies.

There is a story that psychologist Tara Brach tells that illustrates how these two ideas—that we suppress trauma even as our brain changes from it, and we store that trauma in our bodies—intertwine beautifully. A woman recalls being seven years old, and living with her alcoholic father who often beat her. Her mother does nothing to stop him. One night, after her father has attacked her again, the little girl hides in a closet, terrified. She's crying, praying for help. When she opens her eyes she sees a magical fairy who whispers to her that although she can't make all this pain disappear, she can help her to get through it and forget her pain, for now. "I am going to touch different parts of your body with my magic wand and they will change and be able to hold all the terrible feelings for you so that you can survive," the fairy explains. She hides the little girl's fear and rage in her belly.

Another part of her pain she places in her neck. Another bit goes into her chest. One day, she tells the girl, when she is older, her body will begin to hurt. "You won't be able to hold all this in, and your body will start unwinding its secrets." But by then she will be grown and in a safer place so that she can look at the pain she's hidden away. For now she will forget, but later she will remember, somewhere within, that there is a deep wound.

Until then, it is enough to get through what you must get through without thinking too much about it. And get through it alive.

This psychological precept makes sense from a physiological perspective: fight or flight causes our muscles and tendons to tense up. It takes energy to hold on to our pain—we clench our muscles to hold it in, or to hold off the thing we fear. These fight-or-flight stress hormones, over time, up the PIN response and fan inflammation. When we carry this tension for decades eventually the quietly mounting cellular dysfunction and inflammation will erupt in different ways for all of us—chronic illness, depression, body aches we can't explain.

So it makes perfect sense, looking back, that by the time I was in college I was already someplace else, married to my worrying, thinking, planning, anxiety. The habit of mind of living with such negative reactivity had already become who I was, by the age of eighteen.

Even back then—though I didn't yet have the physical signs of it—I wasn't alive in my own skin.

I've gotten to the age of fifty-one living outside of myself, as if the churning thoughts inside my head are my reality.

I don't want to miss living inside my own skin anymore.

Yes, the issues have changed. Now I worry over low white blood cell counts and deadlines and stretching to cover medical bills and if my kids will be okay if something happens to me. The stakes are so much higher.

· 16 ·

The Loss That Lives Forever

"I understand everything that happened to me." I'm sitting in Marla Sanzone's office. She has heard it all from me before. My dad died overnight. My mom had a horrific time, as anyone might. My father's family imploded. I shrug. "I've unpacked all that for years. There's nothing new." What is new, I confess, is the feeling of something heavy and old shifting. The weight of the word *forgiven*. These are like interlinking clues in a crossword—only I'm chewing the end of my pencil, drawing a blank. "What I don't understand is why all this now."

"Perhaps, for the first time, you're feeling strong enough to look deeper," Marla says, echoing what Trish has suggested can happen when we establish a practice of mindfulness.

"But I can't think that there is anything left to look into." Still, I find myself sharing with her the story that Tara Brach tells of the girl who stored her pain away, deep inside her body, for many years, before it rose up again.

"Where do you think you've hidden your pain?" Marla asks, following the metaphor I've offered. Her short, dark hair and pale skin frame large brown and extremely likable eyes.

Her question startles me. We are not being scientific here. I tell myself to let that go. It takes me a second. "You must be thinking . . . in my legs?" I venture.

She settles back in her comfy chair, tucking one foot up beneath the other thigh, as if to say, relax, we have all the time in the world. "What function do myelin sheaths serve?" she says.

"They insulate our nerves. Protect them."

"Protect us and keep us safe?"

I nod, trying to think where she's going with this.

She looks at me patiently. "Did you feel protected and safe when you were twelve, thirteen, fourteen?"

"No, but . . ." I have the uncomfortable feeling that I'm missing something. "Am I not getting it?" I ask.

Her eyes smile. "Our parents are supposed to protect us and keep us safe. But your father disappeared. So he couldn't take care of you. Your mother was overwhelmed. Overnight, you were pretty much left on your own. Unprotected. You were twelve. The parents who were supposed to be there to keep you safe suddenly weren't."

She doesn't go on; she can see from my face that she's connected enough of the dots. "And here I am, decades later," I begin. "And my immune system, which is supposed to keep me safe, has twice attacked my myelin sheaths, which are also supposed to keep me safe." I'm struck by another example. "And my skin . . . ?"

"Insulating, protective barriers that are supposed to shield you and protect you haven't been doing a very good job."

"Problem." I hold up my hand like an emotional stop sign. "My mom had enough on her plate. And . . . I never felt as if my dad abandoned me," I say. I try to dispel the chagrin I still feel admitting my childhood secret. I am, after all, talking to my therapist. "I actually felt as if he were somehow . . . still looking after me." I pause. "Magical thinking and all that."

She tilts her head.

I tell her of how I so often felt my father beside me, in the days and months and even the years after he died. How my grandmother grew worried when she heard me talking to him aloud at night as I lay awake in my room. She thought something wasn't right. But the moments I felt him with me were the only moments that felt right at all, I explain.

"Why do you think he came back to be with you?" she asks, as if what I'm explaining—visitations from the dead—is something she hears every day from those on the mauve upholstered settee into which I've settled myself.

"Well, of course I can't say he really was there," I hedge. "But I . . . felt he was." When I was in high school and college, I tell her, I would sometimes shoehorn bits of science into ideas that I hoped might support the magical thinking of my childhood. Einstein once wrote that death "means nothing"; that those who've "departed from this strange world a little ahead" of us aren't really gone, because the "distinction between past, present and future is only a stubbornly persistent illusion."

I would think of how if, as Einstein believed, energy is neither created nor destroyed but merely changes form, then perhaps my father didn't cease being part of the web of energy that connects us all—his energy just radically shifted into a form I couldn't comprehend. If, as quantum physicists tell us, our view of time and space at any given moment allows us to perceive only one dimension among concurrent parallel universes, then perhaps my dad's death, in that sense, meant "nothing." Even as it meant everything. Perhaps the reality my dad occupied in time and space after his death in some way still intersected with mine, if merely briefly, only I became, like the adults in *The Polar Express*, too grown up to believe, to see, to hear.

These are the sorts of things I would tell myself in order not to punch holes in my own experience.

Later in life I would learn that children's brains often fire up reassuring figures and images to carry them through traumatic years and events. The magical fairy in the closet. The magic sword. The guardian angel. The protector.

"These are the only explanations—or rationalizations—I can come up with," I say.

"When he was alive, you shared a great affinity. A love of writing, books, Shakespeare, journalism, a certain way of looking at the world," Marla says. "You must have felt very validated by him, understood for who you were. Your incredible connection to him was very empowering."

I nod. "Which makes it all the more ironic that I never got to say good-bye." I don't know why I am thinking of that now.

The head tilt again. The steady brown eyes.

"By the time I was allowed to go see him in the hospital he was supposed to be getting better, but he wasn't. He was getting worse; the domino effect of medical errors had already begun."

I explain that for days following his surgery my father had complained of terrible abdominal pain. My mother, a die-hard Scandinavian (her preferred term is *Viking*), insisted on speaking to the surgeon, but he was playing golf that afternoon. The attending doctor filling in told my mother that "abdominal pain after abdominal surgery is normal." She was a little embarrassed. She took him at his word.

I tell Marla all this, eyes leaking, my glasses in my lap. Suddenly my fingers are working like slow, faulty wipers against my cheeks. She hands me a box of tissues.

"And I was of no help. Whether he did or didn't protect me all those years I don't know—but I do know I was no help in protecting him."

"Why is that?"

The trip to Baltimore with my brothers to visit my dad had been prearranged; everyone still expected he'd be getting better that week. Coming home. Any day. But when we arrived my dad was in so much pain he couldn't even bear the motion of the nurse adjusting his bed so that he could be propped upright. He lay against white sheets, his eyes gray as he looked up at his three teenage sons and me. Photographs of the four of us, sailing with him, or from our annual Christmas cards, designed by him to look like newspaper articles about our family misadventures, were taped to the wall across from his bed in his direct line of sight.

I had never seen my father afraid, so I didn't understand the look of fear, and the efforts to mask the look, on his face as he tried to smile at me. Not until much later, when I would feel that same fear while lying in a hospital bed. I only knew that something was terribly wrong. Couldn't everyone see? He wasn't okay. What was wrong with them all? *Why wasn't somebody doing something?!*

Weakly, he asked me for a glass of water. I remember my gladness at being asked to help him, in any small way at all. As if a glass of water might be just the touch, the thing. The pitcher stood on the portable hospital bedside table, angled over his lower body. I picked it up with careful hands. But as I poured the water in the cup my fingers trembled. A large splash of ice water hit my father's lower chest, soaking through his hospital gown. He cried out. A nurse ushered me from the room and told me to wait outside. He needed to rest, she said, gesturing to a place in the hallway where I could wait. I stared out the long, dusky hallway windows, seeing nothing. I don't remember being driven home.

Forty-eight hours later, he died.

Never coming home again.

"I knew," I say. "I knew when he looked at me something wasn't right. Some part of me knew what was happening to him and I didn't say a word. To anyone."

"And you could have saved him?"

"No, I don't really believe that—not rationally," I say. "But if I'd told someone what I saw . . . I should have made someone listen. But no one was listening. Who would listen to me? I couldn't even pour him a glass of water without screwing it up. The last moment I ever saw him he was wincing in pain—because of me." I pause. "If I knew then what I know now . . . I would never have let him go into surgery without the surgeon knowing the medications he was taking. I would have investigated. I would have knocked heads together in the hospital to get some answers."

"No one expects a twelve-year-old girl to save her father," she says. She is quiet for a moment. "Have you been trying to make up since for what you couldn't do then?"

I think of the hours spent interviewing doctors and scientists. But none of it will ever bring him back. Too late for that. For goodness' sake, I think, I am older now than my father was when he died. Let it go, Donna.

"When do we ever just . . . let go of it all?" I ask.

"When we're ready," she says. "But for a long time, not letting go empowered you," she says. "Holding onto the idea that you could have saved him, if only you'd been bigger or smarter or more vocal, allowed you to retain some feeling of power, even after he died."

I am a little blank.

"Feeling you could have saved him allowed you to feel you still had some control over your world. You were able to keep the feeling of empowerment that you would otherwise have lost when he died—because he was no longer there to validate who you were."

I try to let this sink in. But it seems nothing is sinking in. Which probably means it's something I should really pay attention to.

"This is very important," she says. "So I'll say it as often as you need me to. When your father died, you held close to the idea that you possessed the power to change things, to save him. That you could have done something no one else could have done and kept him alive. And that story of your own power kept you alive; it made you feel you could control your world, even as it fell apart, and you lost all control. It served to cover up your own feelings of powerlessness. Underneath the fear that you hadn't saved your father was another deeper, scarier reality—it was just too painful so you covered it up with a narrative that was easier to bear."

I feel as if something thick is being stirred inside by a long spoon. Or maybe dislodged. I'm not sure I like it. In fact I don't.

"When he died, he left you." It seems as if she is talking very fast, though I know she is talking slowly, more slowly than usual. "Alone. On your own. With no explanations. In a world of grown-ups who were either too overwhelmed or too self-involved to notice who you were or to even ask if you were okay."

The room goes a little funny around me. I think of how the year he died I began fainting. In the driveway. The bathtub. Everyone told me to stop being such a drama queen, a hysteric. It turned out, later, that I had such a severe case of vagal syncope my heart was skipping so many beats I'd pass out, see stars, go down, wake up sweating, nauseated. I try to imagine now, not noticing if one of my children was fainting.

"If he loved you beyond time and space, and life and death, if he talked to you and you could talk to him after he died when you were just a twelve-year-old child, well, then you had to be very powerful, didn't you? If you had the power to save him, you must have been quite powerful indeed." She pauses.

I look at her. Something is starting to register.

"The alternative would be to face the idea that he left you alone in a world where no one understood you or watched over you. Where there were no grown-ups to lean on. Where no one even noticed you. With nothing to prepare you to get through without him. No warning. No instructions or good-byes. Powerless."

Another, longer pause.

"If he really, really loved you, how could he leave you like that?"

She is talking from very far away, though her voice seems to be warm, near my ear. "You told yourself you could have saved him because it allowed you to still feel powerful. So powerful you didn't have to face your feelings of how furious you were with him, for abandoning you the way he did."

I realize I've put my head between my knees. I feel engulfed by a big, black, horrific cloud of smoke and bleakness. It eats my air. I can't breathe.

"I need. You. To stop," I rasp.

"You're forgiven, for not being powerful enough to save him," she says, very gently. "Forgiven for not being powerful enough to save yourself when you were twelve."

She is very quiet for a moment before she adds, "And when you forgive yourself for that, you can begin to forgive your father for abandoning you to a painful world. You can stop hiding all that pain deep inside your cells."

· 17 ·

Psychotherapy on Steroids

The timing of the three-day women's silent winter retreat couldn't be better. Or worse. All that time to be contemplative. Too much to contemplate.

The good news is that the retreat leader is Tara Brach. Tara and I have been in touch—by phone and by e-mail—conversing about the search for spiritual wholeness, joy, and well-being despite illness. We've never met, so I'm surprised when we arrive at the same time at the meditation hall and she gives me a big hug. So big that I find myself a little disarmed when she asks how I'm feeling about embarking on my first retreat. I am suddenly confessing to her, without meaning to, that I didn't anticipate I would come to this point in my journey only to discover that I would feel worse.

"Of course you do," she says, without missing a beat. Her long, brown hair curtains her shoulders as she steps back. It may be the color of her eyes, or the vibrant blue pashmina shawl that envelops her, leaving dangling loose corners like tucked wings, but I can't help but think of a delicate, graceful bluebird. "You've come on the journey so that you can contact more of the unlived life, which means unearthing more of the loss you haven't allowed yourself to feel. And, for a time, that feels worse." She tells me that she hears this story frequently. But ultimately, she says, "getting through those feelings is the only way to access the wisdom and joy and belonging you're yearning for."

THROUGHOUT THE FIRST afternoon of the retreat Tara meets with small groups of women. She asks each of us to share, for five or ten minutes, why we are here. What we've met up with in our lives that's brought us to a place where we seek to sit in contemplative silence for three days.

Many women's stories are of physical or emotional illness or distress: pain, disease, depression, and anxiety. They move me, these familiar tales. The young mom who still hasn't recovered from her own abusive upbringing—and who now finds herself impatient and overreactive with her two toddlers and hates herself for her behavior every day. The fiftysomething woman facing her anger over a life usurped by cancer. I understand when she says she is faking her way through every minute of now. The thirtysomething athlete who was in a severe car accident eight years ago that left her with horrific back pain—and who still uses medication just to grimace through each day. The insomniac mother whose twenty-two-year-old son is defusing road bombs in Afghanistan, and who is sick with fear, unable to control the anxiety-ridden tapes that play through her mind every waking hour, of which there are too many.

When it comes to my turn in the circle, and why I have come, I am unobtrusively pinching my own palm to keep tears at bay. Not for myself, but for all the women here.

If my life were conveyed on a map of my world, I say, you'd find me in the center, treading water in a vast ocean, surrounded by shifting continents. The continent of illness. The continent of my childhood: the loss and aloneness, the unfinished business, and wanting to put it all to rest. And the continent of doing, the pedal to the metal day-to-day pressures of my now-life.

Tara nods. I recall her saying, in her welcome talk, that in Chinese script the word for *busy* is the same as *heart-killing*.

These three tectonic plates keep closing in on me, I say, and there I am, very small, desperately treading water, in a large, turbulent ocean, trying so hard just to stay afloat above the chopping whitecaps.

"I feel small," I say. "So very small." This is a simple thing to express, but as I say it I feel very, very sad. Heads around me nod.

"Tell me about small," Tara says.

"I realize that, for a long time, I've been pretending to have a sense of self-power and capability I've never felt."

"And how does that pretending feel?"

"Like a divided life. An onstage life—where I pretend to be this competent person who can take care of anything and is never overwhelmed. But behind the curtain I have this backstage life, where I feel small and unable and overwhelmed. Because of this, I think, I haven't been taking myself seriously—even as I've been pretending that I do."

"And tell me about that—what is the feeling just beneath not taking yourself seriously?"

"Inadequacy. I'm supposed to have all the answers. In my work. For my husband. My kids. Everyone turns to me. No one knows how inadequate I am to the task."

"And beneath the feeling of inadequacy, what's there?"

"Sometimes I'm just . . . angry." I blurt it out, surprising myself. I am not an angry person. But as I say it I realize how true it is. How angry I sometimes feel. How often I am angry with someone for some perceived wrong to me or someone I love. "Sometimes everyone's needs just make me . . . angry."

"And what is the feeling just beneath that? If you were to let those feelings of not taking yourself seriously and inadequacy and anger just burst out of you in every direction all the way out across to the other side of the world, what would be left?"

"I don't know. I guess . . ." I pause. "I think I would be left."

"So," Tara says, "for the next few days you might occasionally drop in the words, 'I'm feeling inadequate, I feel small, I feel angry,' and just allow the experience in your body to be as full as it is. Discover what happens."

. . .

OUTSIDE, THE GROUND is newly covered with our first big snow this year, as if to help shroud us in silence. For the first evening I sit on my hard-back folding chair, a soft, green blanket from home draped over my shoulders, wrapping across my lap. I am alone but together; we are a cocoon of eighty women in this quiet, warm, and dark meditation hall, each looking to get past whatever bleak, flickering thing has kept us from the Life Channel.

I think of a line from one of my favorite books, *The Book Thief*, by Markus Zusak. "Usually we walk around constantly believing ourselves. 'I'm okay,' we say. 'I'm all right.' But sometimes the truth arrives on you and you can't get it off. That's when you realize that sometimes it isn't even an answer—it's a question. Even now, I wonder how much of my life is convinced."

My whole life has been convinced.

I wait. I focus on my breath. The softness of muffled sounds as women around me shift, breathe: their presence.

Or I try. All I can really think about is how much I itch. Not just my chin. My eyelids. Everywhere. My legs. My palms. The bottoms of my feet. I wrap my blanket around me and quietly scratch myself beneath it. My chest. My neck. I can't stop. I try to, but I can't. I get up and go to the bathroom, where I scratch long, glorious red streaks up and down my legs. And then I go back, sit down.

I remember what Tara said. One has to get through those feelings to access the unlived life. I try again. I sit, gently placing my hand over my heart. Each time I touch my chest, the sadder I feel. The more tears leak. The more my gentle touch turns into scratching the skin across my chest. I sit on my twitching hands.

IT IS HALFWAY through the second day before something happens. As with the questions, the answers come, at first, in images.

She is beside me. Myself at twelve. She hasn't yet had her growth spurt. She is small and scared; her legs are so skinny. I am surprised to see that she looks so much like a child. She lays her head on my shoulder. So many adult responsibilities. She is tired. Of being so grown up too soon. A job at the library after school. A bus girl at an Italian restaurant on the weekends. Figuring out what's for dinner. Missing her dad. Telling no one she's afraid.

It strikes me then: much of that description—so many adult responsibilities, telling no one she's afraid—would describe me now.

Here I am, as an adult, trying so hard to be the grown-up. The dog is throwing up; I have a speech to write, a track meet to get to and I don't know the way. I'm so tired and my legs are wobbly, and there are bills to pay, and dollars to stretch, and dishes to do, and dinner to plan, and then I have to catch a train for New York in the early a.m. I don't feel like a grown-up. Not one adequate or powerful enough to handle all the details on top of details and stay calm and kind and alert. I feel like I'm still twelve. Meeting expectations that are over my head. Beyond my ken. Past my stamina level. I'm treading water. Waiting for someone to throw me a lifeline.

It suddenly makes sense to me: the feelings of inadequacy and powerlessness I feel now are the same feelings of inadequacy and powerlessness I felt when I was faced with so much responsibility prematurely as a young girl.

The inability to control illness, financial crises caused by illness, fatigue, the doing without collapsing from the doing. The inability to control my dad dying from illness when he didn't have to, to help keep my mom from collapsing from the doing, the world falling to pieces.

That girl, the girl who lived through all that, powerless, overwhelmed, inadequate to the task of getting through a world falling to pieces on her own—is still traveling with me.

My chest hurts. I feel my chest, my skin, burning like hot iron. My breath comes shallow and short. I focus on filling my lungs, three-part breath—belly, lungs, chest—but I have trouble taking in that much air.

I hold the girl I was, giving her all the love I can.

The area around my heart is spasming. I place my palm against it, the tightness in my chest.

And then I see my sixteen-year-old self, walking toward me, her face long, her blond hair a shield behind which she hides herself. She comes and sits beside me, leaning her head on my other shoulder. She doesn't have to say a word. I feel how alone she is. Brothers gone to college. Dad gone. No more cats at the bus stop. The boats sold. The stars dim. No more laughter. No one has told her why her world has broken to shards, or that, in the end, she will be okay. She rolls her face toward my shoulder.

Twelve and sixteen.

I cradle the two younger me's, these girl selves who are the very ages that my own two children are now. I hug them closer, one on each side, as I have my own kids, time and again.

But then something else happens. Out of nowhere, my brain sends me a kind and wholly unexpected image. A me at age sixty-five or so. A wiser me, calm, kind. More wrinkles. Less fear. She is wearing a beautiful, seafoam blue cashmere hat that one of my best friends knitted for my fiftieth birthday. This older, wiser me places a warm, maternal hand on my forehead, tracing her fingers down the side of my face to gently touch the rash on my eyelids, then my chin. For a few seconds, I feel a burst of relief, she seems so sure of herself.

"You'll see, years from now," she says, her face toward mine, whispering so close to my ear I can almost feel her warm breath. "It all turns out okay. You're okay. You really are."

I am afraid I am going to lose myself in tears. Make a fool of myself in front of the other women sitting near me. But from time to time I hear one of them break into quiet weeping, too.

I recall something I've come across by the famous Tibetan Buddhist teacher Chögyam Trungpa, who was sent by the Dalai Lama to teach in the West. "If we look into our fear, beneath the veneer, the first thing we find is sadness, beneath the nervousness," Trungpa teaches. "Nervousness is cranking up, vibrating all the time. When we slow down, when we relax with our fear, we find sadness." The tears that follow, he tells his students, "are the first tip of fearlessness, and the first sign of real warriorship."

I put my hand over my heart, my twelve-year-old heart, my sixteen-year-old heart. I wipe generations of tears.

"Will I ever get out of here alive?" Sixteen-year-old me looks up at me.

I find myself smiling as I imagine myself stroking her head. "Oh you will," I say. "You will."

I smile at my younger selves. "Guess what you do?" I ask them.

My twelve-year-old self looks up, eyes hopeful.

"You have a wonderful life," I tell her. "It isn't easy." My aware mind considers for a moment, what would I tell my girlhood selves if I could travel back to the world as they knew it? I see myself, thirty-plus years in the past, writing in my journal, telling myself I would become a writer, somehow, even though I was told that that was a silly pipe dream.

"You write," I say. "You really do it. Not just in your journal. You write books and columns and articles and stories." I pause. I know she is terrified of speaking in front of people. I know she lost her voice not long ago while giving a social studies report in front of her seventh-grade class. "You talk to large crowds," I say. "Really." I pause again, realizing that I am not speaking of the things that mean the most to me, or that will mean the most to her. "You have the two most beautiful children imaginable." Both younger selves gaze up at me; it's hard to tell which one is more incredulous. "And they *love* you," I say. "Right now, in this minute, they are the ages you two are now. And I promise you: they will amaze you." I am hit that this is the time—between twelve and sixteen—when everything in my life was bleaker than bleak and I was more alone than I would ever be again in my life. These are the years in my own life now as an adult, with a teen and teen-soon-to-be, when I feel they need me to be my best self. My most competent and wise. They are too old for me to fake it; they see through the cracks when I don't feel well or when I reach the outer limits of my ability to parent mindfully. If you have two teens, you know. They need so much graceful parenting as they make their trial-and-error efforts to strike out on their own. I am not always so graceful. But I am there.

I take in another deep breath. "And . . . you're a good mom." I don't know if I can claim this; so many times I should have been so much more with them than I have been—at the very least so much less annoyed. But my children know in their core that I love them, and they are not alone. Not ever. They get to be who they are. And they get to come to me, and to their dad, when they are afraid or alone or scared and say just that.

They are preapproved.

"And there is one more thing," I say. "You take your time, but eventually you marry your best friend. And the two of you become grown-ups together. You really do it. You create the family you don't have now—for yourself."

The older version of myself, who has been so quiet, hugs us to her. "And it gets even better after that," she says to all three of us. You wake up one day very soon and you love who are. You wake up on your own side."

She winks. I'm wondering, what does sixty-five-year-old me know that fifty-one-year-old me doesn't?

We sit, the four of us. I feel the wisdom of that older, calmer self breathing into me, as I take in each inhale. Filling belly to chest. The old fear, the terrible inadequacy, exiting with each out breath.

And then she, in her seafoam knit hat, smiles, kisses me gently on the forehead, and is no longer there. Perhaps it's not a good sign that my brain needs to send me the crutch of an imaginary, better version of myself to find surety, calm. But I don't care. She has helped me to shore up a little extra strength when I couldn't find it alone.

I FEEL MYSELF expand with the joy of this moment. My sixteen-year-old self looks newly calm, as if she is thinking about the future she is to have, being a writer, being in love, the teenage anticipation she never got to feel because she was too busy feeling afraid and angry and overwhelmed and small. Then, in my mind's eye, they are no longer in my arms; they've melded into who I am. *I will take care of you*, I say, beneath my breath.

And for the first time, I feel something like proud. Proud of everything I've survived. Proud for taking this journey. Proud for coming here, for these three days, to be a warrior on my own behalf.

· 18 ·

Shedding

A week and a half after I get home I go in for a check-in with Rowland-Seymour. I am sitting next to her, by her desk, giving her an update. I tell her about wanting to rip my skin off my body—how the day after the retreat I saw myself in the mirror after a shower and noticed red marks and faint bruises from scratching. Of course I bruise easily, but still.

I tell her, too, about how the muscles in the left side of my chest spasmed for an entire afternoon and evening. She knows that the lead line from my pacemaker box down into my heart is quite old; my cardiac surgeons have wanted to replace it but haven't yet, because the risks entailed in implanting a new lead line have, thus far, outweighed the risk of the old one I have going bad. Of course, a bad lead line probably wouldn't lead to muscle spasms—I'd black out and have seizures. But spasming chest muscles are something you should probably tell your doctor about when you are a cardiac patient.

"Are you still having spasms?"

"Not now, no. Although the left side of my chest is still sore."

She puts away her stethoscope. "I'm wondering," she says. "Were these spasms happening at the same time that your skin was bothering you so much?"

I nod.

"And were you experiencing any shortness of breath or difficulty breathing?"

I had almost forgotten about the feeling that my chest felt so blocked it was hard to take in air. "Yes," I say. "I wondered later if I might be having some sort of allergic reaction; it was that hard to take in a full breath." But, I explain, I was also trying very hard not to sob out loud. Holding back sobs can feel like getting punched in the throat and chest.

She looks at my chin, my eyelids, with her usual professional scrutiny, tilting my head this way and that. She settles back in her chair as if to take me in, all of me. "I don't see any eczema on your eyelids or your chin. There's no redness. No scaling. Have you been using any steroid creams to treat it?"

I shake my head. "Maybe one of my organic all-natural creams is starting to work at last," I joke. But the truth is, I have been stunned, in the past week, that my chin is not puffing up, red and scaly, that my eyelids are flesh colored again, that I can sleep through the night without scratching so much that I find in the morning I've made myself bleed.

"I find this significant," she says. "You've had a highly persistent case of eczema." She leans back over her desk, jotting something down, tapping her pen, then writing something more. She looks up. "So," she says, "let me tell you why I find this so intriguing. In Chinese medicine, grief is related to the area of the body thought of as the 'lung.'"

In Chinese medicine, emotions and health are deeply connected through various areas of the body. But that's as much as I know and I'm not sure what the chest and lung have to do with my skin.

Rowland-Seymour explains that in Chinese medicine, the "lung" is the area of the body directly related to the emotions of grief and sadness, which are said to be integrally connected to the regulation of moisture to the skin, and to respiration. "From this Eastern medicine perspective, when we're imbalanced in the lung—or when we're holding onto our grief or sadness or trauma—we might expect to see shallow breathing, shortness of breath, very dry, itching skin, and skin eruptions."

I am trying to overlay this onto what I already know. "I know that new studies are showing that scratching helps to blunt the areas of the brain that are associated with unpleasant memories or traumas. . . ."

"And the Chinese medicine perspective would tell us that the fact that your skin itched so much and the muscles of your chest spasmed and you felt it hard to take in a full breath—and then it quieted down—this indicates you were releasing a great deal of grief and trauma," she explains.

I think back to those three days in the dark meditation hall. The itching. The grief. The chest spasms. The shallow breath.

"Very interesting," she repeats, almost imperceptibly shaking her head, smiling as if to say, We don't know precisely what's going on and maybe we never will, but this is quite fascinating, isn't it?

"There is one other thing that complicates all this," I throw out. "My own personal biology. As in how genetically sensitive my brain has been to my own experience."

"The sensitivity hypothesis."

"The orchid hypothesis."

"Yes."

I HAVE RECENTLY been reading about a relatively new idea in biological psychology that a few of us—some 15 percent—possess two copies of a variant of a behavioral gene that makes our brain more vulnerable in the face of life's stressors. That same gene—if we have both copies of it—also makes us more likely to thrive in a positive and nurturing environment. Our brain is more plastic, shaped by our circumstances. Some call this the plasticity hypothesis or the sensitivity hypothesis; others term it the orchid hypothesis because of the way this brain plasticity impacts us early in our growth and development. There are children whom researchers think of as "dandelion" children, and those they think of as "orchids." Dandelion children do well almost anywhere, flourishing in any soil whether they grow in the equivalent of a well-tended garden or an abandoned lot. The so-called orchids are more sensitive to their soil, their day-to-day environment. Life's stressors seem to affect them more powerfully.

Orchids possess a variant of a gene called 5-HTTLPR that regulates the neurotransmitter serotonin—which in turn regulates our ability to rebound and recover from serious emotional trauma and distress. This serotonin gene comes in three different variants. The short-short variant—considered the "orchid" expression of the gene—is associated with being highly impacted by one's environment: less able to mange or recover easily from trauma or stressful events—and, on the upside, being more creative, emotionally successful, and happier when shaped by a positive environment. In its short-long expression, the seratonin gene doesn't seem to have much impact. The long-long gene expression, on the other hand, is equated with dandelion-like resilience. Life may be very hard, but one just doesn't seem to feel the pain of life quite so much.

A few days earlier I had a conversation with Srijan Sen, MD, PhD, assistant professor of psychiatry at the University of Michigan Medical School, who recently analyzed over fifty studies to better understand the relationship between seratonin gene variants and increased or decreased risk of depression and illness as adults.

"His meta-analysis showed that the orchid gene variant is correlated with higher rates of depression," I explain to Rowland-Seymour. "But what's really intriguing is that the orchid gene is more likely to be correlated with depression in adults when stressful circumstances occurred in *childhood* rather than when severe stress hits once they're already adults."

The orchid gene, Sen explained to me, plays a far more important role in how well we moderate stress when we are young than it does in how well we moderate stress when we are grown-ups. And, he added, "It may play a direct role in why adverse experiences in childhood affect one's likelihood of having adult illnesses." Let's put it this way: if you possess the short orchid gene variant and yet your life is smooth sailing until you hit adulthood, the job loss or divorce you face as an adult may not make you more vulnerable to illness and depression than those who have the more resilient dandelion gene. But if you possess the orchid gene and hit enough of a rough road as a child, it is a very big deal. It will change your life.

Scientists haven't quite yet figured out all the reasons why. But it seems to have to do with sensitivity to stress. In individuals with the short-short gene variant, researchers have been able to see brain activity differences in how stress lights up their amygdalas. Researchers at the National Institute of Health ran an experiment in which they showed subjects a face that was angry. In those with the short-short variant, the areas of the brain that reflect anxiety and fear lit up more than they did in other participants. They had an increased amygdala response.

When I asked Sen why he thought that kids with the short-short gene variant might suffer from more depression, anxiety, and illness as adults, he directed me back to Michael Meaney's research on gene methylation. It may be that orchid children with the short-short gene variant who feel more impacted by trauma are more likely to undergo the process of gene methylation and stress deregulation. This makes total sense: orchids—whose amygdalas, or fear centers, light up more easily—feel more afraid and vulnerable in the face of threatening traumatic events than their dandelion counterparts who might experience the same traumatic events and feel less anxiety or sense of trauma. As a result, a child with the orchid gene has a PIN response that is more regularly revved up. This makes him or her more vulnerable to the process of gene methylation that fixes the brain in a state in which a floating brain of inflammatory neurochemicals charge through the body—which translates, in turn, into more health risks.

We already know that children with a history of ACEs who also possess the orchid gene grow up to have a greater chance of depression. Young adults with the short-short variant who experienced traumatic childhoods have the most severe symptoms of depression when they grow up. Dandelions do far better. We might extrapolate these depression findings to indicate higher disease risk for orchids in general, because other recent studies show us that long-term emotional distress, beginning in childhood, lays the foundation for ongoing inflammation. Until we have the science in front of us we can't say for sure that orchids who suffered childhood trauma get physically ill more in adulthood than dandelions, but I suspect the answer would be yes.

But the orchid gene also brings with it distinct neurobiological advantages that dandelions don't seem to have. Having a particularly plastic brain also means you have a brain that makes you more responsive to the environment around you in general. The same plasticity of the brain that makes the orchids highly reactive to stress also makes them more easily impacted by what is good in their environment: the love they're shown, the mentor or teacher who helps them, the opportunity to be creative and express themselves—and even efforts to reshape and retrain their brain. When orchid children experience a supportive, nurturing childhood, they actually show the *fewest* signs of depression in later life, even compared to those with the dandelion gene. They become even more likely than other people to develop positive and beneficial psychological characteristics. They do better than dandelions.

Why does all this matter? Growing scientific consensus tells us that efforts to meditate and retrain the brain might help to rewrite bad epigenetics and even induce new, better epigenetics. Undo the damage of gene methylation, or what some scientists now term our "DNA memories." The sensitivity hypothesis, when viewed alongside ACE research, suggests that perhaps those who are most likely to end up facing chronic adult health issues as the result of ACEs are also those who are best able to turn their bad epigenetics into good epigenetics.

No matter who you are—regardless of your experience or your genetics—it is quite possible to engage in regular practices that downshift the fight-or-flight response and grow new, healthier neural and chemical pathways, simply by adjusting your psychological state of mind. Meditation studies in posttraumatic stress patients and others tell us that anyone can get a better brain. And the scientific speculation is that those with orchid genes may have the evolutionary advantage of having the most pliable brains of all.

ROWLAND-SEYMOUR LOOKS THOUGHTFUL. "These are all such important questions to ask, even if we don't have all the answers. But how does knowing all this impact your own journey?"

"I don't know if I have the orchid gene, and I don't really care to be tested for it," I confess. The testing is expensive and hard to obtain outside of a research setting; it's certainly not something the average person could or would do. And Rowland-Seymour and I have agreed that every aspect of my journey should be easy to replicate by anyone, anywhere. "Besides, my genes won't change over time the way blood work might, so even if I did know more about my personal biology, it wouldn't tell me anything about whether my journey has had profound positive effects." I pause.

"But?"

"Some part of me has to wonder if the women most likely to be facing chronic conditions as adults are the women who do have orchid genetics and who faced ACEs when they were younger," I say. "I want them to know that even if they are sensitive and feeling, and came through a lot, although they might sense all that as a handicap, they also, hypothetically, have a leg up."

"And you suspect you might be one of them?"

I smile. "I don't know," I say. "But it's nice to know that if I am, I'm not beyond hope."

REGARDLESS OF WHAT our genetic background may be, our journey is pretty much the same. In the end, there is only one question: am I on the Life Channel? At some juncture in my life, my cells will fail. I don't say this to be morbid, I say it as fact: we are all, eventually, dying—and one day I'll have to find joy and well-being even in the face of imperfect health, no matter what genes played a role in my ultimate demise.

We all will.

What matters is not just whether I've nudged my blood cells this way or that but whether I get back one essential thing: that sense of vital life energy that I haven't felt since I was twelve, standing on my dock with my dad, feeling that surge of aliveness both in the world around me and in my own veins. A sense of excitement about *being here just as we are now*.

I have had that sense of being here since then of course, of being connected to an inner sense of vitality and well-being, certainly—especially when my brain is on love. The dance in the kitchen with my son; talking to my husband as my head lies in his lap; walking down the beach, my daughter's small hand tucked in mine; and many moments more. But this sense of safety and well-being and aliveness hasn't been *who I am*.

Who I feel I really am, at my core, how I feel about what is happening to me—regardless of what is happening—and whether I am connected to the Pain Channel or the Life Channel, will tell me more than any gene or blood test ever will.

PART III

***

Bodywork

· 19 ·

So Why Aren't We All Doing Yoga?

People come to yoga looking for different things. Yogis who, if they were runners would race marathons, tend to be drawn to Ashtanga, or "power yoga." It's fast paced, physically demanding, and athletically intense. If students want to sauna out their toxins while doing yoga, they might be drawn to Bikram, or "hot yoga"—practicing twenty-six strenuous poses in a room that's ninety-five to one hundred degrees. I love the idea of sweating out toxins and have always been a little jealous of friends who practice Bikram, but, like Ashtanga, Bikram is too taxing for the body I have. (I recall hearing someone once say, on the sideline of a girls' lacrosse game, "If Bikram yoga is too difficult for you, the answer is more Bikram yoga!" Bikram yogis are hard-core.) With vagal syncope, a fainting and seizing disorder, which can cause me to faint in saunas, it's out of my range.

Students hoping for a more spiritual practice may be drawn to Kundalini yoga, where teachers wear white head coverings and strive to bring in an aspect of the divine. Poses originate from the base of the spine in order to free energy, or *prana*, from the lower body so it can rise, like the uncoiling of a snake. Anything strenuous at the base of my spine—where disk and sacroiliac joint damage mean I pay for days if I pick up a grocery bag the wrong way—is unattractive. Besides, the people I know who practice Kundalini look great in tight, white yoga outfits. I do not.

Viniyoga is more appealing—you work one-on-one with a guru who takes into account your injuries and full health history. That's more up my alley. But not in my budget.

Vinyasa yoga, a moderately paced practice that involves breath-synchronized, flowing movements that warm up the body, is more my speed. Think sun salutations: swan-diving down, lunging, down-dogging, rising with your arms overhead to the sky. If you can't do a pose, you can take a pause, modify, take your time. I like the idea that in my yogic effort to activate the healing potential of my brain I am greeting the sun rising over the horizon, the whole wide world—if only in my imagination, from my little, green rubber mat. Iyengar yoga is another option that appeals, as well it should: it was developed for people with injuries and health constraints. Teachers use props—blankets, straps, blocks, and chairs—to make sure a student's body is properly supported and aligned to get the maximum benefit without injury.

Happily, Vinyasa and Iyengar are both found in what's termed hatha yoga. *Hatha* literally means *yoga*. Hatha yoga is the forefunner of all ancient postural yoga practices. Today the term refers to a general hatha practice in which the goal is to find harmony and balance among mind, body, and spirit. The poses, or asanas, are usually basic, slow, and controlled, and are accompanied by breathing exercises, or *pranayama*, which emphasize stress reduction, relaxation, and a meditative state. Hatha teachers often walk around the room giving fine-grained instructions, adjusting body alignment, reminding you to pay attention to your breath, to what's happening inside as you stretch and strengthen at the same time. And to be mindful as you move of what you can and cannot do.

That sounds like the best of all yoga worlds to me.

AND THAT'S THE beauty of yoga. Those of us who can no longer do the types of exercise we used to can often succeed at some form of yoga, in some way.

Still, there are, as with any form of exercise, drawbacks. If we try to do spinal twists and balancing poses that are inappropriate for our body, we can dislocate disks and pull muscles. People do. Which is why it's so critical to be realistic as we try to match our physical state and ability to whatever yoga style we choose. Second, although yoga is a unique and powerful form of exercise, it is not aerobic; it doesn't provide us with the important cardiovascular benefits that come with running, interval training, or vigorous sports. Which is why I still head out for long, brisk walks—in addition to my multimeditation dog strolls—walking so fast that I break into a sweat. If my body would allow it, I'd add a spinning class or jog a few miles for a true aerobic workout—high-intensity cardiovascular exercise lowers blood pressure and protects against heart disease. But efforts to spin and run have, in the past, simply led to more injuries. Still, I can't pretend that yoga—especially when practiced as safely and slowly as I must—will give me the cardio benefits we all know are important.

Having said that, if our limitations are what bring us to yoga practice, well, that may be to our lifelong advantage. Neuroscientists are just now fully grasping the profound ways in which yoga helps to activate the healing responses of the brain and establish a positive feedback loop between state of mind and cellular vitality. As it turns out, the overall positive mood benefits of practicing yoga are more robust than what we see with other well-studied types of exercise. For instance, women who take a twelve-week class in yoga show greater improvements in mood and lowered anxiety levels than do women who expend the same amount of time and energy walking. That's saying a lot—because, for a long time, walking has been the all-around wonder exercise for those of us with chronic health constraints. At least, that's been the case for me.

Yoga, even gentle yoga, it turns out, offers so much more.

Fibromyalgia patients find their pain, fatigue, and overall mood significantly improve when they practice gentle yoga poses for eight weeks. They're also less likely to worry over and "catastrophize" the pain they do feel. The same is true for breast cancer survivors who take part in an eight-week yoga class. They feel less fatigue and a greater sense of "emotional well-being" compared to patients in a control group. Their pain lessens as their mood grows more positive. Six months of yoga reduces fatigue in people with multiple sclerosis; lessens disability, pain, and depression in adults with chronic low back pain; lowers disease activity in patients with rheumatoid arthritis; and improves allergy symptoms. Cancer patients who practice yoga report significantly less anxiety, depression, and stress levels as they manage their disease.

What strikes me most about these studies is the frequent mention of the relief patients feel from anxiety—even while engaged in a practice that brings them face to face with their physical limitations and vulnerabilities. We've talked about how important this is before. When you're wrestling with a chronic condition, much of the static on the Pain Channel is the reaction we all have to straight-out pain, but a good part of it is also the worry that attaches itself to our experience, bringing with it a whoosh of inflammation-bearing fear, courtesy of the negative floating brain. Fear makes pain loom larger than life—and the Life Channel. A muscle spasm in my leg to me is painful, but if I begin to worry that it's the familiar first sign of demyelination and GBS taking over my body all over again, my whole being pulses with live-wire, neurologically sparked fear that shoots through my central nervous system like emotional kudzu. I start to feel eerie twitches of pain in my calves and legs that I wasn't aware of a moment or two before. The sensation grows. It's as if my thoughts and fears of pain have caused another layer of pain.

What surprising new research tells us is, in a sense, that's exactly what's happening: I'm sending those pain signals to myself.

When we're injured or feel a symptom flare, nerve fibers send "danger signals" to the brain. The brain makes a rapid decision as to whether these pain signals are worth getting all worked up about—or not. And the thing that makes the brain decide one way or the other is whether or not we, personally, perceive that specific pain to be a threat. In other words, you might stub your toe and expect the pain to fade after you count to twenty-five, because your parents always told you that's what happens when you stub a toe. You've stubbed your toe hundreds of times before. And the pain always subsides. And so it does this time as well. Your brain isn't paying all that much attention; there is no perceived threat.

But let's say you have a history of fairly severe arthritis and your left hip suddenly begins to ache, right after you get out of bed to turn off your alarm. The ache seems sudden and deep and new. Moreover, its onset reminds you of when the pain in your other arthritic hip first began; the one for which you're currently considering a hip replacement. Your brain is suddenly ultra attentive to the danger messages now emanating from your left hip. Fight or flight—the PIN response—kicks in: *What's up now and how much is it going to hurt?*

The sympathetic, or stress-now, nervous system gears up for battle. As the SNS kicks in, neurons fire and old neural networks are activated—based on your past memories and experiences—which remind you of other potential threats. You might suddenly think of how when your grandmother started to have pain in both hips she was in a wheelchair five years later. Or that when your other hip first started aching you missed two weeks of work and you're pretty sure it cost you your promotion.

Now you're really under threat. It's an ever-expanding threat—it's not just your hip. It's your future, your independence, your mobility, your job, your finances. The brain begins to add up all these potential perceived threats; danger impulses multiply, and pain amplifies.

For someone else, the same level of pain in his or her left hip might be perceived as a two on a scale of one to ten. It's an ache—like a stubbed toe—that will surely dissipate. But because of the perceived threat this same pain represents to you—and to your brain—for you it's a seven out of ten. It really, really hurts. It's scary how much it hurts. The pain isn't imagined. It's quite real.

We think of physical pain and emotional pain as being two separate things—but they aren't. The brain regions involved in experiencing signals of physical pain are the same brain regions involved in our perception of emotional pain.

Which brings me back to yoga. Regular practice of yoga dampens our self-reactivity to both physically painful and emotionally stressful stimuli. Here's an example: researchers took fifty healthy women between thirty and sixty-five years of age—half of them regular practitioners of yoga who had been doing yoga one or two times weekly for the last two years and at least twice weekly for the last year. The other half were "novice" yogis, who had had about six to twelve yoga sessions, tops. Researchers put everyone through physical and emotional stress tests, including immersing the women's feet in extremely cold water for a minute, after which they were asked to solve a set of increasingly more difficult math problems without paper or pencil. Participants' inflammatory cytokines—which whip up the stress-now system—were then measured.

The results were astonishing: those who had very little yoga experience, the "novices," had inflammatory cytokine levels of IL-6 that were 41 percent higher than the yoginis who had practiced regularly for two years. The regular yoga practitioners came into the study with lower levels of inflammation than the novices, and they were also better able to limit their stress responses than were the novices when faced with physical and emotional threats.

There are several ways in which yoga slows down our sympathetic nervous system and activates the healing responses in the brain at the same time that it helps us to grow physically stronger and more resilient.

One of these has to do with a particular type of chemical in the human brain known as GABA—short for gamma aminobutyric acid—which is essential to proper brain function and also promotes a state of calm. Low GABA levels are associated with depression and anxiety disorders. In the study comparing those taking a three-month yoga class with those doing a walking program that required equal physical expenditure, women who practiced yoga showed higher increases in GABA levels as compared to the walking group. Even one yoga session can significantly raise feel-good GABA levels in the brain in those who regularly practice. For this group, even a single hour of practice can yield a 27 percent increase in GABA levels—with some yoginis showing an increase as high as 80 percent.

The yoga brain is a calmer brain, offering us more long-term mood protection than other forms of exercise.

Another reason for yoga's profound benefits is the way in which yoga seems to help increase blood flow to areas of the brain associated with healing. Practicing yoga for three months has been shown to increase the cerebral blood flow to the parts of the brain that help us move toward a feeling of well-being—and decrease blood flow to the areas of the brain that Velcro us to bad thoughts—the areas we'd like to quiet. PET scans on yoga newbies before yoga training and after show significant decreases in the cerebral blood flow to the amygdala—that old reptilian fear center—and increases in blood flow to the frontal lobe and prefrontal cortex. The prefrontal cortex, as we know, is the area of the brain that's responsible for problem solving, emotional clarity, helping us to mediate between conflicting thoughts and make choices between right and wrong and good and bad. It helps us to overcome our older reptilian brain urges, which tell us to eat too much, or put sex before love, or scream at someone, or lie to get what we want. The prefrontal cortex is the brain center from which springs our better self, our sentient being, and the habits of mind and behavior we engage in through its neuronal fire-wiring define, over time, our personality and our sense of a greater consciousness.

But one of the most significant reasons we see so much change in our mental outlook with yoga may have to do with the unique way in which yoga breath combined with how we stretch and tone our muscle tissue in yoga poses work in tandem to send neurological signals to the brain that alter—and better—our emotional state.

We know, from previous research, that our emotional state of mind affects the rate, depth, and pattern of our breath and vice versa. Manipulating the breath in ways that match up with a range of different emotional feelings can account for as much as 40 percent of the variance in how much we feel a particular emotion—be it anger, fear, joy, or sadness. Think of gasping in pain, sighing in relief, holding your breath in fear.

When we combine yoga breath inhalation and retention with

physical poses that open up, align, and mechanically stretch our body tissue and muscle, we send signals to the brain that bring down the PIN response in ways other forms of exercise just don't replicate.

Yoga poses help to strengthen weak muscles that are critical in allowing us to fully engage in the type of slow-rate abdominal and diaphragm-based breathing that can bring about powerful neurological changes. For example, one of these forms of slow breathing is what yogis call *ujjayi pranayama*, or "ocean breath." This form of breathing involves inhaling and exhaling through the nose, first filling the lower belly, bringing the breath to rise into the lower rib cage, and finally moving upward into the chest and throat. It's a breathing technique almost identical to the "three-part breath" practiced in both meditation and yoga—but with an "ocean breath" sound added by moving the glottis (think snoring) and narrowing the throat passage so that the breath makes a rushing sound as it passes in and out. As yogis work to control the breath they are simultaneously—whether they realize it or not—working the diaphragm, strengthening it, stretching it. The more they practice the breath while holding a pose, the more this toning and stretching creates greater muscle strength and allows for deeper, slower breathing. And the greater the impact this breathing has on the neurological signaling that enhances the parasympathetic nervous system's activity, bringing us to a calmer state of mind.

This signaling takes place through the most important nerve in our body, the vagus nerve, which travels from our brain stem all through our torso and serves as the parasympathetic nervous system's message pathway for carrying information from brain to body about pain, temperature, heart rate, blood flow, blood pressure, breath and respiration, and gut sensations. The vagus nerve also does something else pretty stunning: it helps to provide stability to our body's immune response, calming down the inflammatory reflex that plays a role in almost every disease from cardiovascular conditions to rheumatoid arthritis.

The physical change toward slower, rhythmic breathing, combined with positioning the body and mouth in specific breath-friendly postures, and muscle stretching and toning, stimulates the vagus nerve to send signals that inhibit the sympathetic nervous system's pathways. And this, in turn, leads to a slowing of brain wave activity causing the overall switch toward parasympathetic—or positive floating brain—dominance. After having allowed our sympathetic nervous system to dominate us most of our lives, we give our parasympathetic nervous system—the purr-now system—the upper hand.

This long-term physiological switch toward "parasympathetic dominance" effectively "resets" the autonomic nervous system, calming us, and changing our physical experience of pain, both in the present moment and for the future.

Two researchers, Patricia L. Gerbarg, MD, assistant clinical professor in psychiatry at New York Medical College, and Richard Brown, MD, associate clinical professor of psychology at Columbia University, have recently published a number of papers investigating how stimulating the vagus nerve and parasympathetic nervous system through yoga breath work helps to build stress resilience. They make the excellent point that "although many medicines can temporarily dampen the sympathetic system, including antianxiety drugs such as valium, and some antidepressants, there are no medications we can take to boost the parasympathetic nervous system." Yet simple, gentle stretching and slow yoga breath practices—free and available to all—can potentially "strengthen and recharge the parasympathetic nervous system rapidly and effectively."

In a recent controlled trial, Gerbarg and Brown found that a two-day training workshop on breath techniques helped patients with inflammatory bowel disease to boost their parasympathetic nervous system activity. Patients' levels of inflammation decreased and, in some cases, says Gerbarg, "they experienced healing of their chronic GI lesions." Breath practices, she emphasizes, can "activate the parasympathetic nervous system acutely, often within five to ten minutes." Yoga is not just preventive medicine; it's restorative. Yoga not only revitalizes our cellular health in both brain and body; it changes the brain in a preventive and protective way—so that when we come up against stressors and pain, we're more resilient, less reactive, and more likely to send forth a positive floating brain than a negative one, allowing the healing feedback loop to remain in motion, and even become our new default setting.

OF COURSE YOGA is also exercise. And as such, it offers us most of the powerful healing benefits of exercise in general. Indeed, neuroscientists have only recently come to understand the ways in which physical activity in general enhances the healing responses of the brain. When we regularly exercise, we bring regenerative life into every existing cell in our bodies—including our brains—literally creating entirely new cells for the very first time.

Until quite recently, neuroscientists believed that the brain stops producing new nerve cells, or neurons, at birth, and thereafter the roughly three trillion brain cells we're born with begin to dwindle slowly and predictably away. We drink too much, fall off a horse, or simply turn another year older and we lose more brain cells, which can never be replaced or renewed. But that long-held scientific theory has, in the past decade, been replaced by a new body of game-changing findings.

In one more example of the brain's elegant intricacy, it turns out that small populations of immature nerve cells dwell in our adult brains well into old age. In a process scientists now refer to as neurogenesis, given the right cues, these immature nerve cells can divide and differentiate into either new, baby neurons, or they can become additional neural stem cells that integrate into and enhance the brain's neural network. These new neurons often come to life in the areas of the brain associated with higher learning.

As we age, however, these neural stem cells tend to become less able to transform. They're there, but it's as if they've shut down and aren't responsive; think of them as being in something akin to a cellular coma. They aren't getting the cue that tells them to wake up.

This somnambulant state is caused by a protein found throughout the body known as bone morphogenetic protein (BMP), which inhibits cellular development. The more active BMP is in your brain, the less responsive your neural stem cells become, the less neurogenesis occurs, and the less vibrant your brain, your thinking, your state of mind, and your ability to learn new things.

Exercise awakens these quiescent neural stem cells. Exercise in general influences the rate of neurogenesis as well as the survival of new neurons after they are born, and it does so through multiple pathways. To give just one example, when we exercise we increase another protein, what we might think of as one antidote to the BMP-induced cellular coma, appropriately named Noggin (yes, Noggin). The more Noggin you have, the less BMP is able to suppress undifferentiated cells and keep them in twilight sleep. The more neural stem cells divide, the more neurogenesis you undergo. Brain activity becomes more vibrant and alive because there are literally more active brain cells to go to work. Exercise profoundly stimulates the production of Noggin and the division of undifferentiated neural stem cells into new neurons in the brain.

Remember how yoga has been shown time and again to relieve anxiety, worry, and depression in the chronically ill? There are clear links that suggest that physical activity in general—and we may assume this includes yoga—helps to relieve depression and move our state of mind toward well-being explicitly through the process of neurogenesis.

Researchers have long hypothesized that major depressive disorder is related to a decrease in the synthesis of new neurons in the brain, and that antidepressants increase the production of these new, healthier neurons. They came to this realization in part based on one striking fact: the time it took for antidepressants to kick in and relieve emotional symptoms in patients dovetailed with the exact same amount of time it takes for neurogenesis to occur, and for new neurons in the brain to become fully functional.

As it turns out, this time lapse is the same for exercise. It takes an identical amount of time for exercise to activate new neurons in the brain as it takes for antidepressants to kick in and start making us feel better by activating new neuronal growth. In a recent evaluation of a number of studies that show physical activity to be an effective treatment for depression, strong support emerged that the reason for patient recovery was, indeed, adult neurogenesis. And experts believe that yoga in particular may facilitate the potential for the brain to undergo these neuronal changes.

PHYSICAL ACTIVITY ALSO helps generate stem cell growth and individual cell repair throughout the entire body. In animal studies, exercise increases the number of stem cells in muscle fiber by almost half. This increase in muscle stem cells makes rats more likely to demonstrate what researchers refer to as "spontaneous locomotion," that feeling that signals our body to just get up and dance.

A little like rats whose brains are on joy—or whatever the rat equivalent to joy might be.

When we engage in physical activity, we also wake up something within our cells called mitochondria. Often referred to as the power generator of our cells, mitochondria combine oxygen and nutrients to create cellular fuel, which translates into fuel for our bodies. As we age, the number of mutations in our mitochondria accumulates to the point that our cells stop being able to make the repairs they need to stay healthy. Our muscles get smaller; our brain volume shrinks. Our hair turns salt and pepper. We start to look and feel old. Our cells literally become frail.

Physical activity combats the mitochondrial dysfunction that accompanies aging and boosts mitochondrial robustness. In one humorous study, well-exercised mice didn't undergo the changes in fur color that are analogous to our hair turning gray as we age.

There is one other fact I like knowing, because I am not a rat but a woman managing a set of chronic illnesses. Women under stress who exercise have longer telomeres than women undergoing chronic psychological stress who don't exercise. It helps to know, too, that just fifteen minutes of physical activity a day reduces our risk of death by 14 percent and increases life expectancy by three years. Being active reduces frequency and severity of colds and our risk of Alzheimer's.

As someone with my share of neural damage—from stress-reactive tracks I've laid in my adult brain as a result of my history of ACEs, missing white matter due to GBS-related myelin damage, and the Velcro-to-the-bad tracks from our universal evolutionary biology that we all share, the idea that getting up and moving my body in vigorous ways can create brand-new neurons to help redirect the old neural tracks I'd rather kiss good-bye—that has my attention.

A Gentle Start

When I ask a few people in the meditation community—many of whom are yogis—whom they would recommend to lead me safely into a yoga practice despite my many years of physical therapy, I hear the same name: Stan Andrzejewski. He will often work with students with physical injuries to help them safely get ready for a yoga class—and because he is a physical therapist, my insurance covers it.

Andrzejewski, who owns one of the oldest yoga studios in the Greater Baltimore area, has the white-cropped beard of a yogi and the full, pink cheeks of an enthusiastic child. He's brought both that wisdom and energy to his work, combining what he's learned as a licensed physical therapist over thirty-eight years with his twenty-six years as a yoga teacher. In addition to teaching the art of yoga as physical therapy, he specializes in working individually with students with orthopedic and neurological issues. When we first meet and I tell him that I hope to find a way to "work around the many things wrong with me," he admonishes me with a smile. It's clear he's heard this before and doesn't like broken-body thinking. "Your movement vulnerabilities aren't to be 'worked around,'" he says. "We want to relieve them and provoke change with timely, skillful posture and movement through yoga."

Stan watches my unskillful posture as I stand, walk, and bend. He surprises me when he tells me that much of my back pain—which I've assumed to be entirely disk related—is due to my sacroiliac (SI) joint inflammation. The way I usually stand—slouched, with one hip jutting out, my weight on one leg—a stance that echoes all those years of carrying a baby or toddler on my hip—just keeps sparking more inflammation. It jams all my weight down on that SI joint, inflaming it, when what I want to do is relieve pressure and let the inflammation die down.

Most of us have some sort of posture problem, Stan says, and if we correct it, we can relieve a significant layer of our physical pain. I'm surprised that mine is so dreadful; my mother really did have me stand against a wall with a book on my head when I was very young, I tell him. After a while I got so good at it I could keep a copy of *Five Little Peppers and How They Grew* flat on my head while setting the table.

Stan smiles, cocking his head to one side so that his white beard juts out, elflike. "Clearly, that was a very long time ago and things have changed." The good news, he says, is that there are poses and stances to correct the damage I've unwittingly been doing every day, which retrain the spine and give it a chance to heal naturally.

"Every time you bring your legs to your chest, rest in child's pose, go into a downward facing dog, or do a soft forward bend, you're providing relief for your SI joint and giving the tissue a chance to repair," he says. He asks me to practice, as I go through my day, imagining that there is a large rubber ball in the center of my torso, and it's rotating in an upward motion from my pelvic bone toward my waist, causing me to pull in and tone my abdomen, at the same time that it's relieving pressure on my sacrum. Stan is a master of images—and I like that. I can work with that.

I imagine the blue, rubber ball rotating up over and over. The image brings me an awareness of my stomach muscles firing up, strengthening, toning, and protecting my back muscles, all the while relieving the pressure on my SI joint. Stan wants me to concentrate on that image as I practice *tadasana*, or mountain pose. "Bring your weight evenly into all four corners of your feet and lift your toes," he says. "Now rock front and back, side to side, feeling the four corners of your feet, pressing a little more into your back outer heels for stability."

My feet are so close together that I expect to lose my balance, and for a moment I do teeter, but somehow concentrating on what's happening in the ball and heel of each foot while I lift my toes keeps me more connected and grounded into the floor. I wobble but I don't fall down.

I am not falling over, and I am not being held up.

My GABA levels are on the rise; my vagus nerve is stimulating my parasympathetic nervous system to quiet my stress response and, as with all forms of exercise, I am, I like to think, stimulating those first stirrings of neurogenesis, awakening my cells. We don't have all the answers yet as to when and how these moment-by-moment cellular changes happen in real time. But this opening up feels like self-administered cellular medicine, no doctor's appointment required. I feel lighter on my feet. Stronger in my base. Something like a soft, tingling energy travels up and down, between the crown of my head and my toes. It's a little like opening a bottle of sparkling water.

For the next week, as I stand in line at the post office, watch at the sidelines at Claire's lacrosse games and Christian's track meets, and wait for the woman at the health-food store to tally up my groceries, I practice my new stance. I find I'm not tired while standing; I'm not scouting for the next chair or that acceptable piece of dirt on the ground on which to sit. Standing, breathing, rooting down, growing taller. It feels like . . . strengthening some core within that is more than muscle deep.

Day by day, a small layer of low-grade pain that I've learned to live with for years in my back, my pelvis, my sacrum, even my legs, begins to lessen. Its disappearance shocks me one morning when I get out of bed. I am used to waiting during the first ten or fifteen minutes of the day, as I go through my morning routine, for the cranky, creaky pain to subside in my left back and hip. Like the Tin Man in want of an oil can. I have learned to wait, too, for any numb body parts—an arm I slept on, a foot that's still dead—to come fully back to the land of the living. Yet as I groggily head downstairs to make my first cup of green tea, it dawns on me that I'm not wincing over my back or my left hip. Numbness—well, that's a perennial. But the back and hip pain are . . . not there. Noticing this one change makes me think: I also haven't been wincing when I get up from the couch or out of the car. I realize, as I kick off my slippers and stand in *tadasana*, watching the hot water course over my tea leaves, that I hadn't realized how much those small aches were adding to my Pain Channel static until I see what I'm like when just this one small symptom fades into the background. An hour later, when I get into the car to take the kids to school, I slide into the seat and twist to buckle myself in without the usual small flinch. I can't help but smile. Can the simple adjustments I've made lead to a change that will lift a layer of pain away—all through my day? And so quickly? Apparently they can. Later that day I read a little more about the research on the benefits of practicing simple yoga postures: even short-term "yoga interventions" are proving to be remarkably helpful in patients suffering from back pain.

The next step, Stan tells me, is to engage in a gentle yoga class and work toward skillfully grounding, centering, and lifting my body. An inner and outer steadiness. He has just the teacher: Julie Madill works well with injuries and special needs, though I somehow doubt she has seen too many folks like me.

· 21 ·

Oh to Be a Yogini

I have been wrong before (ask my teenagers) and I am certainly wrong this time. The women unfurling their mats around me are not in designer yoga gear. Julie Madill's class is full of forty- to seventy-something women who have been through breast cancer, hip replacements, and carpal tunnel surgery. They are veterans of what Stan calls "movement vulnerabilities."

At the beginning of each class, Julie calls out to her students, who seem, many of them, to have become as familiar as girlfriends. "Anything new or different going on? Louise, how is that wrist? Carrie, how are you feeling? How was that treatment last week? How are we all feeling today?"

And the thing is, every woman shares. And that, really, is because Julie Madill is sitting in the front of the class, listening, nodding, taking our collective pulse. After just a few minutes of murmuring and sharing she seems to get an overall gist of the energy meter of the dozen or so women before her, and she decides exactly how we will spend our next hour and a half only after assessing the subtext of what we've brought her on that particular day.

What surprises me, during the first few weeks I take her class, is that everything we bring her is okay. On a day when I walk in feeling muddleheaded and so energy deficient I'm teetering on the verge of wanting to spend the entire class lying prone, and wondering if, in fact, maybe I should roll up my mat and just head out before I embarrass myself—well, it turns out that many of us are feeling that way.

Julie has a long history of her own health challenges. When she was eighteen she was in a car accident and broke her back—her injury still flares up to this day in recurring spinal fractures. She's dealt with the "emotional burden," she says, of a chronic autoimmune skin disorder, known as vitiligo, which causes visible pigment discoloration, for as long as she can remember. And in the process of having and raising her four now-grown daughters, Julie has managed "severe" postpartum depression. For many years, the pain of a ganglion cyst—a tumor over the top of a tendon in her wrist—caused debilitating tendonitis, impacting her practice. Like so many of us she's racked up her share of injuries as an active woman over fifty: a sprained sacrum and pelvis, a mild concussion, a dislocated kneecap, and a tear in her right shoulder.

In the course of classes, Julie will sometimes hear a student talk about a sore shoulder or knee surgery and say, "I know, it's really hard," and we know she does know. She gets down on her mat and shows us exactly how to protect ourselves if we have that particular vulnerability and what the work-arounds are. Often, she's played with a pose at home with a student in mind until she's figured out precisely how it can be done safely, and she demonstrates for us all.

We usually start class with toe and foot stretches to warm up the feet and move on to hip openers and hamstring exercises. Once Julie has slowly—stealthily—brought us through enough poses that we begin to feel the slow, inner churning of our vital life energy, or *prana*, we stand.

What amazes me is that no matter where I start when class begins, and even on those days when I'd like to slink home, unseen, I'm always ready by the time we come to our feet, to stretch, to move, to breathe.

It is in these moments of standing poses I am reintroduced to parts of my body I didn't know were waiting to greet me again. I become intimately acquainted with what my limbs can and cannot do. We practice our sun salutations, rising up, arms spread wide, arching our backs into a supported, standing back bend, our hands guarding the base of our spines, then folding into *uttanasana*, a standing forward bend. As I fold in two, my hands dangle toward my calves. I tell myself it doesn't matter if other women around me are more flexible and can touch their ankles, or even reach the floor—but I peek. Quite a few can. I'm not sure what I would have to do to bend over that far, but I think it would involve tumbling unprettily onto my head.

We rise slightly up while still bending forward, creating a flat back, parallel to the floor, then fold toward our toes again before sending our feet to the back of our mats in a downward-facing dog. I have a perfect view of my longish legs—one I would never get any other way. *You jolly old legs, just look at you*, I think. This, I quickly decide, is my absolute favorite pose. No one can bother you in a down dog. I can't even bother myself. I can't see anyone or anything but the peaceful, soft, quiet world beneath all of the demands, shoulds, and coulds that bark at me day after day. When I am in down dog there is nothing before me or behind me, just here, now, the effort to enter fully into the demands of the pose.

Julie likes lunges. And we do a lot of them. Which makes class interesting, because when we are lunging and it's time to switch and bring our back foot forward, I have a little problem. I can't swing my left foot forward to the front of the mat, to where it needs to be between my hands. I have to physically pick it up and place it on the spot where I want it to be. I have to do the same thing when it's time to bring my right leg forward. Still, once I get used to doing it, it doesn't seem so bad. And I am probably not alone. Which is why Julie sometimes says, "If you have to pick your ankle up and move it, that's fine too," as if she is one step ahead of me in my own head.

One day I find myself, while dragging my ankle forward to switch legs in a lunge, muttering, "I'll never be able to bring my foot to the top of my mat." Julie hears me, her head swinging in my direction. "Never say never!" she calls out.

As we move, Julie teaches us about muscle energy. "It's easy to just hang out in a pose," she says. "I used to try that all the time when I first started. You just kind of stay in position, looking like you're engaged, but you're just waiting for the pose to be over, for the teacher to say, 'Okay, up you come.'"

I wonder, as she says this, if she is looking at me. We are lunging—did I say she loves lunges? I am thinking: exactly how long am I going to have to do this? Because my muscles are quivering so intensely, it feels as if everything that connects me together inside is about to shatter like glass at the sound of a high pitch.

"When you just 'hang out' the pose is much harder to hold," Julie continues. "It hurts. Your risk of injury is much greater." If you want to make a pose easier, she asks her student friends, "What do you have to do?"

A chorus: "Use muscle energy."

"Yes, muscle energy," she repeats. "Ground your right leg into the floor, firing up your quad, and extend all the way through the back of your left foot, right through to the back of the room," she instructs, her voice conveying the energy she wants us to utilize. "Feel your core energy as you lift your torso and come into a back bend. Open your heart. Draw your shoulder blades onto your back. Relax the jaw. Breathe." Mind you, we are still lunging.

My thigh shakes and shakes. Julie reminds us, whenever we struggle to hold a lunge-based pose—and this may be why lunges are among her favorites—that the psoas is often called the "fight-or-flight muscle." I have read this, too. The psoas is the only muscle that connects our lumbar spine to our legs. As it passes the abdominal cavity, it supports all of our internal organs. When we feel a sudden sense of fear, worry, or loss, our psoas tries to protect us from physically or emotionally falling prey by clenching and firing up. It ignites so we can flee or stand our ground or kick out against whatever enemy we feel we face, even if it's an apparition of the mind.

When we have grown up with a lot of adversity, or ACEs, our psoas takes the big hit. The psoas subtly and silently stores all that emotional trauma, holding to it tight for decades, even a lifetime. When we're in a searching-for-tigers-in-the-bushes state of mind—as we so often are—we prime the psoas in anticipation of the next bad thing. Our body wants to release that muscle tightening and return to a state of homeostasis through physical exertion, effectively metabolizing our excessive stress hormones by fleeing as fast as we can or striking out to defend ourselves. The natural conclusion of fight or flight is to expel that physical tension in physical ways.

But because we don't release that physical tension and stress, we never reach that natural conclusion. We walk around in a state of contractedness day after day. We get a little tighter. Less flexible. We're in more pain. We can't let go of what bugs us. We hold it all in our muscles, and nowhere more than in our psoas.

The more we keep feeling the fight-or-flight, or PIN, response, and don't resolve that cycle through physical release, the more trauma the muscle holds. The more we hold.

Lunges release the psoas. They release us.

As my thigh shakes it sometimes seems as if all that pain and fear that's been held tight inside all these years—fear of people I love dying, fear of being paralyzed again, fear of falling not just on my face but in life—is vibrating, slowly, out so that I might become stronger not from sheer, imposed will and determination, covering up the truth of who I am and where I've been, but with a new core, an inner strength. Longer telomeres, new neurons, stronger mitochondria powering up my cells.

And I think that if I can bring in my calming breath, my mindful thinking, when in truth my quad muscles might spontaneously combust beneath me, I can bring in calming, focused strength anytime, anywhere. Everything seems more possible.

I HAVE BEEN training with Julie for several months when one day I find, as I try swinging my left foot forward to the front of my mat, that I am able to bring it just shy of where I need it to be without a physical assist. From there I can shimmy it forward. It's not easy; it requires focus. But I can do it. There are other changes, too. When she asks us to "jump, hop, or walk" both feet forward as we move from down dog to *uttanasana*, or standing forward bend, I no longer penguin-waddle my feet to the front of the mat. I jump. I feel a little giggly the first time I do it. I barely cover half the distance I need to. Like a frog not quite making it to the lily pad. But the thing is, I jumped. Something I haven't been able to do in a decade.

A week or two later I notice, as we fold forward in a sun salutation, that my fingers are brushing not my calves or my ankles but my toes. As the tips of my semi-numb fingers sweep over the tops of my semi-numb feet, the nerves in my toes jingle jangle a little, sending tingly nerve sensations up my legs, as if I've brushed sensitive piano chords that respond to the slightest touch. Julie asks us, if we can, to circle our fingers and thumbs around our big toes. I hold them in my fingers, gently, firmly. My oft-broken, numb big toes. I can almost feel the life breathing back into them. I am humbled by the sense of coming full circle, beginning to connect back to my own body, after so many years of pretending that this physical self was just a banged-up vehicle, a broken-down car that would always let me down and never take me through a single day without running out of gas, and my having to pull over to the side of the road.

Now I get it. Yoga puts gas in my engine. This is what it feels like to raise the GABA levels in my brain, to promote neurogenesis, to rev up my cellular mitochondria. This is cellular rejuvenation. I feel it, pulsing through me, buzzing, tingling in my fingers and thighs and nose. My toes.

That day, at the end of class, after having rested in *savasana*, as we sit cross-legged, Julie asks us as she always does to end with one *ommm* together. My *ommm* is long, and hearty, and glad. Not over any one specific happening or event. Just glad. Generally, wholly glad. I can't remember when, really, I felt this glad.

· 22 ·

Body Love

As I use my body as my test kitchen, I notice more changes. I'm feeling more capable as I take care of small, routine, physical tasks. Just this morning, I put a heavy stack of Pyrex bowls away on a high cabinet shelf, and it didn't seem so much of a Herculean effort. Often, I leave heavy bowls and pots for Zen to wash and put away. But today I did it. I took in a deep three-part breath, stood on my tiptoes, and I did it. My toes didn't give way. And my arms didn't sag for those residual, post-exertion, rag doll–like moments I've grown so used to.

I'm curious—mindfully so!—about what this small lift in energy might mean I'm able to do. Can I get more physical? Try something more? Riding a bike? Ocean wave jumping?

But I have gotten myself into deep trouble thinking this way before. First, I'll simply try doing yoga a little more often.

Sometimes that means just doing a down dog beside my desk, to clear my head. Or a ten-minute sun salutation. One day, when I can't find the quiet state of mind I need to think through whether to take on a potential tricky work project that's come my way, I go into warrior pose. The answer comes to me.

Working more yoga poses into the small moments of my day does something else. I'm sitting less. I sit down, usually, far too much, both driving my kids to and fro, and working at my desk. Remember those rats in the lab that were filled with "spontaneous locomotion"? That desire to just get up and dance? Yoga has jump-started in me a need to keep moving my limbs. Being stationary or static for too long feels wrong.

And the fact that I feel the inner call to move is very good because sitting down, as it turns out, is very, very bad for your body and your cells.

FOR MOST OF human history, we lived life in motion, fleet on our feet. We gathered fruit, eggs, nuts, and hunted bison and small game. Getting enough to eat took up much of our day. The closest we came to sitting was to squat beside the fire as we roasted our dinner.

It's only in the last few relative milliseconds of human history that we've sat through each day, commuting to jobs by car or train, spending eight hours at our desks, sitting down again once home, slaves to e-mail and TV. We're plunking ourselves down more than ever before in human history—an average of 9.3 hours a day—more time than we spend sleeping.

Sleeping is restorative. Sitting is the opposite. A woman who sits just six hours a day is 40 percent more likely to die within fifteen years compared to a woman who sits less than three hours a day. People who sit for most of the day are 54 percent more likely to die of a heart attack. In fact, people with sitting jobs have twice the rate of cardiovascular disease as people who stand while they work. The engineer who drives the train has a shorter life span than the conductor taking the tickets. People who sit and watch TV for three hours or more a day are 64 percent more likely to die from heart disease. And each extra hour of TV you watch adds up to an 11 percent higher risk of dying.

The shocker is that these differences are even seen in individuals who regularly exercise.

Here's why: sitting down for just two hours causes very bad things to happen in your body; it causes your good cholesterol levels to drop 20 percent. Electrical activity to the legs shuts down. (This helps me to understand why my post-GBS legs so often go Gumby when I'm sitting and writing, or meditating; my solution is simple: rub the dogs' tummies, one foot for each pup, to keep my muscle nerves connected.) This lack of electrical activity into the legs leads to a domino effect of negative metabolic effects. Our level of C-reactive protein, an important marker of inflammation, rises. The rate at which we burn calories slows down to about one calorie per minute. The enzymes that help break down fat drop by 90 percent. Which may be why sitting more is a health-risk behavior that leads to obesity, heart disease, and earlier death. When a certain enzyme, called lipoprotein lipase (LPL), is decreased for long periods, as it is when we're sedentary, our bodies no longer efficiently break down fat in the bloodstream and convert it into energy.

Why is this biological cascade so damaging? LPL enzymes break down our lipids and triglycerides, sucking fat out of the bloodstream. When they aren't doing their job, levels of our high-density lipoprotein, or HDL (good), cholesterol fall precipitously. When we sit, the muscles that help us to stand lose 75 percent of their efficiency in removing these bad lipoproteins from our bloodstream. After four hours of sitting on our behinds, the genes responsible for regulating glucose and fat begin to shut down. Over time, this loss of cellular efficiency adds up to a shortened and far less healthy life span.

Even a regular exercise practice can't undo the deleterious effects of sitting too much and too long.

Which means that we have to do two things at the same time: sit less in order to prevent these negative cellular effects—and exercise enough to kick in the positive process of neurogenesis.

If I am going to sit less, I want more of my nonsitting time to be spent doing yoga. I already take both of Julie's weekday morning classes, and weekday mornings—right after the kids go to school and just before I start my workday—are the best time frame for me. I'm not sure how to find another great yoga fit.

• • •

LATER THAT WEEK, I get my answer. A yoga teacher named Mira Tessman turns out to be our substitute teacher at our meditation *sangha*, filling in for Trish. I have met Tessman before; she taught a yoga class during the Tara Brach meditation retreat I attended over the winter. I first noticed Tessman in the retreat meditation hall, as she sat in the quiet sea of women—before I knew she was to be our yoga instructor. I sat off to the right, in an area set aside for those of us needing folding chairs for our legs, our backs, our private aches. Whenever I looked across the room from my higher vantage point, I took note of her sitting grounded and tall on her meditation cushion, her dark layered hair and blue and gold shawl falling softly over her shoulders. My brain dimly registered, for reasons I couldn't explain, that here sat a welcoming heart with a vibrant life energy—perhaps because just the sight of her across the room somehow made me feel calmer.

A day later, when I attended Tessman's yoga class at the retreat and met her, I understood why she gave this impression. In addition to being a certified hatha yoga teacher for the past few years, Tessman has also been a practicing psychotherapist for the past nineteen years. In the yoga class she taught, she wove these two healing philosophies together by asking us to drop in self-reflective questions while exploring poses. It was inviting. Still, her physical pace was a little too vigorous for me. I fell over once and had to sit out a few of the poses toward the end. I wonder if now I could safely handle her class. After our meditation *sangha*, I ask her to tell me a little bit more about the local community yoga class she teaches—I want to be sure it's not too much for me.

"It isn't a gentle yoga class. But there are lots of women there who bring an intention for healing and growth to the mat," Mira says. "They do only what they can. I think you'll fit right in."

The next day I e-mail Mira for directions to the community class she teaches. It turns out it's not far from me. I tell her, too, that I'm curious about what brought her, as a psychotherapist, to practice yoga. We arrange to meet at her office.

She carries so much yogi-calm that I'm nonplussed when Mira, who recently turned fifty-seven, tells me, as she prepares two cups of tea, that it is only very recently—over the past twelve years—that she's managed to rise above a lifetime of depression.

And that transformation took place on a yoga mat.

Mira grew up the oldest of six children on the border of Texas and New Mexico, near El Paso. Her father juggled three jobs to make ends meet. She helped clean house and take care of younger siblings—often feeling, she says, "like my mother's slave." Mira could leave the house for school but coming home too late from playing hopscotch with the neighborhood kids could get her a slap in the face. She spent her days trying to keep up with her mom's demands—and sometimes keep her siblings away when her alcoholic father hit her mother.

In high school a journalism teacher took note of how bright Mira was—especially for a girl from the "non-college-track" side of town— and mentored her along. By the time she left high school she'd become the editor of the school yearbook and was enrolled in the local university.

But she was still living at home. And nothing there had changed. Desperate to get away from the hands of her raging and controlling father, she married a man she knew she probably shouldn't in the way distressed girls sometimes do just to get the hell out. Her husband to be was moving to Maryland—and getting far across the country was no doubt part of the attraction. Her little brother sobbed, begging her not to leave him. She felt she had to or she would be trapped with no way out.

But her husband, not so surprisingly, turned out to be a ramped-up version of her own father; in the year after their wedding he sometimes beat her in an alcoholic rage, the way she had seen her father beat her mother. One night he was so drunk he pinned her down on the floor and held his hands around her throat. "My life flashed before my eyes, just in the cliché way they say it does," she recalls. Suddenly, miraculously, it seems to her now, he passed out on top of her, mid-punch, dead drunk. It took her almost an hour to slowly maneuver out from under him without waking him from his stupor and make her way, deadly quietly, injured and bloodied, to the door. She spent that night on the floor of a nearby shopping mall, where a guard found her, carried her to his truck, and got her medical attention.

"My self-esteem was in the toilet," she says, almost forty years later, as she lifts her mug of tea, steam curling around her face. I struggle to see the beaten-to-an-inch-of-her-life girl inside the woman who sits before me, her face broad and tan, the small diamond stud in the crease of her nose winking in the light from the window. "I was deeply depressed. I was desperate to somehow get back to college. I couldn't get past all the trauma, all the years of feeling like I didn't matter. I felt so much shame. Inside I couldn't have been any smaller."

After escaping her marriage, Mira reenrolled in a Maryland community college. In order to meet a physical education requirement, she took a dance class. "When I was moving my body I felt alive, I felt joy, expressing myself that way." But her dance teacher told her that her hips were too large to ever perform.

It was crushing. And it was a gift. "So I switched to yoga." Her dark eyebrows dip and widen as she gives a half smile, and I have a fleeting image of an eagle's wings spreading.

At first, Mira merely took note that on the days she took yoga class, she felt better. And for a very long time, that was that.

Fast-forward twenty years and she was remarried—this time to a remarkable partner. She had been to college and grad school and was now a licensed psychotherapist with a busy family life, raising two children. On paper, at least, it seemed she'd performed a life makeover of epic proportions through utter will and determination, rising from living on the financial edge and amid neglect and abuse to finding financial security and a loving family life. But inside, she says, "life felt really difficult, like I was always swimming upstream against a hard current, always exhausted. There was no joy." She was still deeply depressed. "I had been married for years. I had wonderful children. I had been to college and grad school and had a successful practice and a very supportive husband," she remembers. "I'd made all the right life choices. But I still experienced the world as a gloomy and terrible place and nothing ever felt right and I didn't know why."

She recognizes the irony, she says, that as a therapist who helped pinpoint clinical depression in others—despite how "successful" she might seem to the world around her—she was in so much denial about that suffering within herself. "I didn't have an official diagnosis," she says. "But I knew. And my husband knew. I made life miserable for everyone around me, especially myself." One day her husband flat-out said, "You're depressed; you're in denial, and you've been in it for too long. I love you but I'm at the end of my rope. I can't live with this. You have to get help."

That wake-up call a decade ago—from the man she loved and didn't want to lose—first led to antidepressants, which did elevate her mood. Too much so. "I felt so good that nothing concerned me anymore," Mira recalls. "I was lost in la-la land." She gained thirty pounds, morphing from a size eight to a size fourteen in three months. "I let so much roll off my back that some days I would get a call from a client saying they were at my office, and where was I? I'd never bothered to write the appointment down."

She weaned herself off the medication—and fell off the precipice. It was difficult just to get out of bed.

Then she remembered how moving her body in yoga had once made her feel. She started to go to a yoga class once a week. Every time she rolled up her mat after class she felt better. So she started to practice every morning, in her bathrobe, before she went to work each day—"even if only for five minutes." She signed up for a more advanced yoga class that was tough—so physically demanding it pushed her to her edge, to a place where she had trouble just hanging on to her emotions.

"On the mat, I would find myself fighting my demons," she says. "You're not good enough. You'll never be good enough no matter how you try." Mira's teacher was tender and supportive when, during the quiet minutes at the end of yoga class, as students rest in what is known as *savasana*, or corpse pose, those feelings of loss and worthlessness would rise up in her, and she would burst into quiet tears. Often, Mira would still be lying in *savasana*, weeping, after the rest of the class had filed out. "I would just grieve and sob. And as I did I felt this shift, this energy moving through my body like a wave—what I think of now as *prana* grief—waking me up, slowly washing out my pain."

She is quiet for a moment and then goes on. "Over time, I began to realize that all that swimming upstream against the flow didn't have to be so hard, that there was a better way."

I look at her across the table and tell her, "I know." I wrap both hands around my warm teacup. "I know exactly how that feels."

She smiles. "I had a feeling, or you wouldn't be sitting here."

After her youngest child left for college, Mira signed up for training to become a yoga teacher. At fifty-three, she was the oldest student taking the course. "The next oldest person was ten years younger," she recalls. "I had to work hard to set aside the small, critical voice inside that kept yelling at me that I was too old to be a yoga teacher, that my time had come and gone. I kept going."

She feels humbled and privileged when she's teaching, she says, to be in the presence of a "community of people who, like me, find that when they come to the mat they don't have to pretend to be who they aren't. We are who we are, right here in our own self-truth." Mira believes, she tells me, that sometimes "the dark cloud of depression or pain we feel becomes a comfort zone. We get so used to it that it becomes who we identify ourselves to be. Yoga invites us out of that comfort zone so we can meet the dark cloud for what it really is and move out from under its oppression." This is really what our *tapas*, or sacred heat, is, she tells me: disciplining yourself to hang on that edge of a challenging pose, even when you want to give up, until you discover a resource, a strength, a vital energy inside that you didn't know you had. That vital energy comes out into the body and into your awareness. You begin to own that energy in a new way and take that ability to finally be comfortable with whatever is true for you off the mat and into your life. "This awakening on the mat leads us to authenticity and true aliveness, which brings us joy. It's a gift to be in the midst of witnessing that transformation take place for people."

THERE IS A Buddhist saying that we should "take the fruit of the path as the path." In other words, if we want to walk toward healing, then we must practice what heals. The practice itself will be the road that takes us to our destination. A Native American proverb puts it a slightly different way: if you want to know where you're going, look where your feet are taking you.

My feet keep taking me back to the mat.

At the beginning of each class Mira asks us to "connect with the intention that brought you here onto your mat today. Inside each of us, there is a small seed. Ask yourself, 'What is it that I want life to give me, what do I want to create with my gifts, how do I want this seed to take root within?'"

I hear it, my prayer for myself, "May I grow into a person of joy. May I be so joyful that I bring this joy to others."

Mira works with us frequently on balance poses. Dancer. Tree. Eagle. Sometimes I fall over. The neural signals that should be racing down to the soles of my feet for balance aren't connecting; some of my axonal nerve damage that makes these stances so difficult, I know, will never repair.

But over time, some other connection clicks in. As if the subtle realignment from the crown of my head down is enough to cause my left leg, left ankle, the ball and heel of my foot to stay "bolted to the floor," as Mira puts it. I improve by tiny degrees. As we go into tree pose, I raise my right foot off the ground for two seconds, five, eight. And I think back to those endless months, not so long ago, when I was unable to get to the door of my own bedroom on my own two legs. Lifting my toe, damaged as it may be, and standing on one foot, is a monumental thing, no matter how brief.

One Friday morning, I find myself making my way through one yogi push-up, or *chaturanga dandasana*, without falling to the floor, before arching back up into the relief that is down dog. The next week it is two. It is a victory. For weeks, whenever I tried to lower my chest so that it hovered between my hands, without letting my breast touch my mat—I found myself collapsing, slapping down. Then, one day, I can do it. Hold myself up. I send Mira silent gratitude for pushing us to work on tough, weight-bearing poses—holding long squats in goddess pose, practicing *chaturanga* over and over. I like knowing that when we practice these and other weight-bearing yoga poses we lessen our risk of osteoporosis. That in addition to spurring on new neuronal and cellular growth I'm building better, stronger bones. But there is a deeper feeling, a feeling of *I can*. And that expands inside me to a feeling that *I am*.

To move my body and like moving it, to reconnect with my body without fear, to fall in love with the feel of my body moving in space—an eagle, a warrior, a half moon—this is what I have been after. I remember hearing once that the composer Chopin, tired by years of being ill, confessed to the writer George Sand, "My earthly body has been a terrible disappointment to me." I get that. I have lived that disappointment.

To love my body as I once loved it when I was very young, before life fell to pieces, racing my brothers as we swam across our creek in the Chesapeake Bay, the sunlight golden on their wet, flopping hair, our retriever paddling faithfully beside us, jumping through the grass in a sack race at the March of Dimes fairs we'd put on, sailing my tiny little dinghy and pulling the jib in tight as I hiked out, moving closer against the wind.

To feel myself that strong again. Even if I can no longer swim hard, jump high, hike out. Simply to feel that inner active glee again, movement inside of the body I have now.

To be a body of joy.

The Life Force

One day, in an evening class I attend of Mira's, held at her office studio, we practice laughter yoga. For the first few minutes we do simple exercises, practicing the art of what's called gradient laughter, faking laughter until it gathers momentum and turns into the real, hearty thing. We pretend to throw our smiles at each other. We touch our fingertips to our noses and go *ho ho ho* and *he he he*. We stick our elbows up and out to our sides and walk around the room pretending that we are blowing up imaginary party balloons. We *ha ha ha* and *ho ho ho* when we are done and wave good-bye to our balloons as they whiz through the air.

I catch myself feeling self-conscious, and tired—it is eight o'clock on a Thursday night—wondering if I'm doing it right, if my every *ha* and *he* and *ho* is more mechanical than everyone else's. Mindfulness, ever my ally, kicks in. *Thinking. Judging. Forgiven.* We hold an imaginary cell phone to our ears and laugh as if the person on the other end is telling us the most hilarious thing in the world. The sight of six women doing this in one room turns out to be funnier than I would have imagined. The woman I'm facing, who I know is recovering from breast cancer surgery, breaks into a spontaneous, natural laugh for the first time. Seeing her laugh makes me happy. It's contagious. I can feel my laugh start to undergo its "gradient" change—from canned to genuine.

We pretend to open our credit card bill and burst out laughing as we look inside and see the bottom line. Each time we finish an exercise we put our thumbs up in the air, smile, and call out to each other, in unison, "Very good! Very good! Yay!" It's funny to congratulate a room full of grown women as if they were little kids who just took their very first steps.

We each take a partner, move to hug her, and pretend to be shocked, springing away. Suddenly everything we do strikes me as funny. A laugh generates up from my diaphragm, and the more I laugh, the more laughter erupts. Mira is laughing as hard as any of us. It's a high. It's time for class to end but we can't stop laughing. We are laughing too hard. I am a laughter balloon, high, free, whizzing around the room as the laughter frees me.

I float out the door and into my car.

I REMEMBER READING once that Oprah Winfrey sent her "resident skeptic" to a laughter yoga class to find out if it was just hype and hot air. He came back and said as he sat on her show, "A stress lifted from my soul. It lifted from my body."

I can relate. It's one more tool in the toolbox, like mindfully sighing, loving-kindness meditation, and down dogging, to lift me out of myself when I need it most.

Which is probably why we often suggest someone "laugh off" a stinging remark. Laughter puts an immediate buffer between what's happened and our emotional reaction to it. It helps us to see situations that appear to be threatening or overwhelming in a more realistic light, dissolving paper tigers into thin air.

Around the globe we all laugh in the same pattern—*ha ha ha*—whether we speak Mandarin, French, English, with one-fifteenth of a second "ha's" repeated every fifth of a second. I wonder if we evolved with a universal *ha ha ha* to counterbalance our evolutionary propensity toward chemical reactivity.

Laughter quickly activates the area of the ventromedial prefrontal cortex that produces and floods us with feel-good endorphins, simultaneously deactivating the amygdala. A hearty guffaw relieves physical tension and stress from our muscles, leaving them in a state of relaxation for a good forty-five minutes.

All this, in turn, helps to improve the function of blood vessels and increase blood flow, protecting against heart disease, lowering inflammation in patients with diabetes, combating depression, protecting the immune system, and improving the quality of life for breast cancer survivors.

In one recent study, just watching thirty minutes of a comedy film, *There's Something About Mary*, caused study subjects' arteries to expand, whereas watching a stressful movie, *Saving Private Ryan*, caused arteries to restrict 30 to 50 percent. If we merely think about watching a humorous video, we reduce our stress hormones by more than a quarter. We also up our levels of human growth hormone, which helps to boost immunity and reduce anxiety by nearly 90 percent.

But what's most helpful is that laughter brings about these physiological changes whether the laughter is genuine and spontaneous, or self-induced at will. The brain doesn't distinguish between authentic and faked laughter. Within a minute or two the same benefits begin to take place within our cells. Psychologists recently compared the effects of three potentially mood-improving behaviors on a group of university students. They had the students try forced laughter, faking a smile, or howling. Forced laughter boosted mood far more than faking a smile did. Howling, just for the record, did nothing for mood at all.

A FEW EVENINGS later, my family starts to go to the dark side—a meltdown over a lost homework paper that somehow segues, don't ask me how, into who last walked the dogs and who left their dirty dishes on the coffee table. I feel the edges of a premenstrual headache. A maternal fatigue and frustration start to gather steam inside. . . . I fake a smile that could, because it is not real, morph into a maternal howl. As in "*How* can you expect me to do everything?!" I think of the science and, fake smile glued on as a temporary stepping-stone toward the real thing, corral my recalcitrant teenagers and cranky husband and pair the family up in twos. I promise an extra slice of the hot (gluten-free) apple pie that's in the oven if everyone will pretend they are blowing up laughter balloons and letting out giggly air.

But, of course, as we are a family with children, the exercise quickly degenerates into certain people pretending to make sounds as if they are letting out another kind of air. Call it whoopee-cushion humor. Nevertheless, within three minutes there is a great deal of laughter, so much laughter that Christian is doubled over, then laughing on the floor with Claire and the dogs, which are smiling, too, as dogs do. The homework turns up magically a few minutes after. It seems a glorious spring full-moon night to walk the dogs, and everyone decides to take a study break for fifteen minutes and go. The dirty-dish culprit puts them in the dishwasher. A family of four with its prefrontal cortexes high on endorphins. Amygdalas quieted. My head, which a few minutes earlier usurped all of my attention, suddenly feels entirely fine.

I don't know who starts it, Claire or me, but one day I find that she and I have adopted a new habit. When one of us is really irritable, we start a laughter contest. We stand just about nose to nose with the maddest, angriest face we can muster until one of us cracks. I always lose. I always laugh first. But really, either way, I win. I am laughing with the girl I love most on the planet and we cannot stop laughing together.

THE NEXT WEEK, on Friday, when I go to Mira's morning class in the church basement, she turns our attention, as she sometimes does, to exploring the yoga breath. We often practice *ujjayi*, or ocean breath. But today, as we come up into mountain pose, she teaches us Kapalabhati breath, a yogic breathing technique thought to send waves of energy through the entire central nervous system, invigorating our brain, cleansing the mind. Some refer to it as "skull-shining breath."

We take in an initial long, deep breath, then push the air out through our nose in short, sharp exhalations. Each rapid exhale causes our body to pull more air back into the lungs, Mira tells us. Our lungs fill up by themselves from the vacuum formed by emptying them during our forceful exhalation. It's a superfast breath—so fast that at first it feels impossible—especially while concentrating on standing in mountain pose. My first thought is that I sound like a woman panting in childbirth, or a locomotive train huffing up a hill. Only Kapalabhati breath is more rapid. Concentrating on forcing out the rapid exhale at the same time that I hold my mountain pose with integrity takes every bit of concentration I have. And then I realize I am doing it. I am breathing air in while only concentrating on my exhale.

My skull does feel shiny. A little high. And then we transition out of Kapalabhati. We move into a slow and gentle three-part breath, allowing the body to cool down, and feel the tingling effects, the yoga afterglow.

I'VE READ THE science on rapid versus slow yogic breaths. It's intriguing. Although we tend to assume that when we breathe fast we are filling our body with more oxygen, that's a yoga myth. In reality, our red blood cells, which contain a protein called hemoglobin that soaks up oxygen and spreads it throughout our body, really don't carry any more oxygen to the bloodstream no matter how fast or slow we breathe. We can bring more oxygen into our body by engaging in aerobic exercise and getting our muscles moving and our heart rate up—but not by manipulating the breath per se. That's a yoga myth. What really happens in yoga breath is a little different. When we practice the slower three-part and ocean breath, we're getting our feel-good effects, as we've seen, by stimulating the vagus nerve and helping the parasympathetic nervous system to dominate. With rapid breaths such as Kapalabhati breath, something completely different occurs. We start to feel lighter in the skull because we're literally changing our body's carbon dioxide level.

Richard Broad explains this complex finding very well in his recent investigative book, *The Science of Yoga*. When we start to breathe fast, blasts of fresh air with "extraordinarily low concentrations of carbon dioxide rush into the lungs" lowering our body's level of the gas. Our body tries to compensate by drawing the carbon dioxide in our bloodstream out and into the lungs. This shift in carbon dioxide reduces the flow of oxygen in the brain. Think hyperventilation. Think fainting. Researchers have found that fast breathing cuts levels of oxygen in the brain by as much as half. Which is why, in Mira's class—perhaps especially given that we are women of a certain age—we practice Kapalabhati breath in very brief and short cycles, moving after just a minute or two into our rhythmic ocean breaths again.

AS WE TRANSITION through ocean breath into warrior pose, in a row of women wall to wall, it hits me that almost all the women in this group are older than I am—perhaps by at least a decade. And yet they are stronger and more flexible than I am. As we get older, aging takes so much from us. But yoga seems to give us so much more, even as we gray.

That day, after I leave class, I wave to the road workers who have cordoned off part of the road to traffic. When I do they do a double take, unaccustomed to such a friendly smile. Several people are honking—the light is green and no one can go. Two workmen wave back. One blows me a kiss. I laugh. He laughs. He turns his sign and shows me the SLOW side and waves me forward. I wave to the honking car behind me. I think of a quote Mira has shared, from yogi TKV Desikachar: "The success of yoga does not lie in the ability to perform asanas but in how it positively changes the way we live our lives." Something is changing inside me. It's not just that I'm manning the gates that hold back my ruminating thoughts better. It's something more. I'm drinking less poison. I'm having fewer of those bad, mad ruminating thoughts. I'm not thinking *Why are they fixing the road at rush hour!* in the first place.

As I drive I fall achingly in love with a bank of clouds stitching white and bursting and round along the horizon, as if they are staring right at me, saying: *Look at us! Look up here!* All around me, the spring buds are bursting on the trees. The pink and plum and white blossoms shimmering amid a sea of green take my breath away.

The Oldest Medicine

The first known record of acupuncture as a healing art appears in an ancient text dating back to 200 BC, known as *The Yellow Emperor's Inner Canon*, a medical guide structured as an ongoing dialogue between an emperor and his court physician. Then, as now, acupuncture is based on the philosophy that placing needles along key meridians in the body awakens the body's own invisible healing force, or qi (pronounced chee), encouraging that qi to move. As our own inner qi is freed to travel up and down our body, it clears energy blockages that have led to—or been created by—illness, injury, fatigue, anxiety, depression, past trauma, or ongoing daily stressors.

For centuries, Westerners assumed acupuncture was little more than voodoo medicine, ranking somewhere in effectiveness between bloodletting and snake oil. But as Western medicine has become more sophisticated so has our ability to investigate whether and how acupuncture might actually change the biological pathways of both body and brain on a cellular level.

It turns out that twenty-two hundred years after this medical technique was first described in ink, many of the 365 key acupuncture points used by the emperor's physicians to awaken qi correspond to muscle trigger points—or nerve bundles—"discovered" by modern-day researchers. Acupuncture meridians often run along the same major arteries and nerves that pertain to the organs for which they were originally named in ancient China. The "heart meridian" runs up across the chest and down the left arm—the same path that pain radiates down when someone experiences a heart attack. The "gallbladder meridian" corresponds to where a physician might expect to find a gallbladder patient complaining of a pain he or she can't explain— emanating all the way up to his or her upper right shoulder.

Devotees argue that acupuncture's longevity, coupled with a body of studies showing its clear benefits, is ample proof of its efficacy; others point to a controversial new trend in the research showing that the plusses of acupuncture may stem from little more than the power of placebo.

Research seeking to quantify the medical benefits of traditional acupuncture has exploded in recent years. The Mayo Clinic recently reported that acupuncture relieves symptoms of fibromyalgia, easing pain and significantly combating the fatigue and anxiety that can accompany fibro symptoms. Women with polycystic ovary syndrome, or PCOS, show lower levels of the testosterone that contributes to their symptoms and experience more regular menstruation when treated with acupuncture. For women with PCOS, acupuncture is a more effective therapy than exercise. Acupuncture is proving to be a better treatment for lazy-eye syndrome in children than the traditional approach of "patching"—putting a black eye patch over the strong eye to help strengthen the weak one—a process I well recall enduring as a nine-year-old child.

But most of the research on acupuncture has focused on how powerful a tool it is in the arsenal of pain management.

There is a story in my husband's family that bears this out better than any study I have ever read. Twenty years ago my father-in-law, then head of surgery at a city hospital, decided to investigate acupuncture as a healing modality. He traveled from New York to Los Angeles to his native Japan and trained with the top practitioners in the world. He came home to his Baltimore hospital to continue his surgery practice, meanwhile completing his course work in both medical acupressure and medical acupuncture. Soon after he implemented an informal study to see whether performing acupuncture on surgical patients would help with his patients' post-op recovery. The results, he told us at the time, were so profound that he found his acupuncture-treated patients were feeling better and more symptom-free in half the time he and the hospital staff would normally expect. His patients showed, he said, "noticeable energy and resiliency." He decided to "abandon the knife" and open a full-time medical acupuncture practice—in hopes of preventing people from ever having to arrive in the surgeon's office or hospital in the first place. He didn't need to read the next twenty-some years of data about to emerge on how acupuncture significantly relieves pain, reduces nausea, and increases feelings of well-being to convince him of what he already witnessed at his patients' bedsides. He wanted to get busy. He wanted to help more people feel better faster.

So it's no surprise to my father-in-law or to other long-standing medical acupuncturists that recent MRI research shows exactly how acupuncture changes the pain-processing centers of the brain and helps to promote healing. When study participants are made to experience physical pain—yet receive acupuncture simultaneously—regions of the brain involved in moderating our perception of pain become more active, reducing the degree of pain we actually feel. Similarly, when researchers press very warm heat against a study subject's skin, receiving acupuncture lessens the level of pain he or she experiences. Not surprisingly, acupuncture has been proven time and again to be a dependable treatment for lower back pain.

There are a number of hypotheses about ways in which acupuncture might work to relieve pain symptoms. Researchers at the University of Michigan Chronic Pain and Fatigue Research Center recently illustrated how acupuncture increases the binding capacity of a particular neurotransmitter system known as mu-opioid—or painkilling—receptors. When activated, these receptors help to dampen pain signals—including those generated in the fear-and-pain-activating amygdala.

This intrigues me. These same mu-opioid receptors are crucial in determining our overall state of mind. Mu-opioid receptors regulate the function of brain regions that help modulate what psychologists call positive or negative affect—meaning whether we experience a positive sense of joy, a keen interest in the world around us, and an inner well-being, or veer toward a negative set of emotions such as anxiety, sadness, anger, and depression. When mu-opioid transmitters are deactivated in the amygdala and other brain centers, we feel more negative feelings. Upswings in the activity of the mu-opioid receptor system usher in a state of well-being, joy, and a sense that all is well with our world—what we have been calling the Life Channel.

Stimulating the mu-opioid receptor system, then, appears to be directly linked to turning down the volume of the Pain Channel. And acupuncture appears to be a simple, risk-free way to operate that control dial at will.

But acupuncture works through more than one biochemical pathway. One group of investigators recently injected mice with an inflammatory substance and then gave the mice the equivalent of acupuncture for thirty minutes to see if it helped to relieve inflammation. It did—more than a little. Levels of a powerful natural enzyme produced by the body called adenosine, known for its anti-inflammatory properties and role in pain management, increased twenty-four-fold in the tissue fluid surrounding the acupuncture needle site. Injected mice given acupuncture had fewer pain symptoms than mice that were injected but didn't receive acupuncture.

Other studies are stacking up showing that acupuncture is a successful treatment for conditions including pain, fatigue, nausea, irritable bowel, carpal tunnel syndrome, headaches, infertility, asthma, arthritis, and depression.

Nevertheless, there is growing speculation that these advantages can by and large be reproduced with placebo, or "sham" acupuncture. One study will appear showing that traditional acupuncture is as efficient as medication for relieving nausea, and another will appear a month later showing that acupuncture is no more beneficial for nausea than a sham placebo acupuncture treatment.

Take a recent study looking at cancer patients being treated for nausea. Patients were divided into three groups. One group was given real acupuncture. A second group received placebo, or sham, acupuncture, a procedure in which patients think they're getting needles inserted into their skin, but instead blunt, telescopic placebo needles are merely pressed against the skin's surface at the same key points that needles would normally enter. A third control group had a standard care regimen. Both the patients who received genuine and sham acupuncture experienced significant relief from nausea—but those receiving standard care did not.

It's a confusing picture. So confusing that a number of research institutions have been busy trying to tease out if traditional acupuncture and sham acupuncture are truly equally effective in promoting healing in patients and, if so, how their benefits might differ.

Their findings are instructive. As it turns out, real and sham acupuncture differ a great deal and in important ways—and the benefits each provide new insight into how we heal.

Recent examinations via PET scans and MRI show a measurable difference in the brain's active response to real acupuncture versus superficial, or sham, stimulation. While real acupuncture with needles excites multiple brain and chemical pathways—stimulating the opioid system and endorphins, increasing positive affect, modulating pain centers, and downshifting the amygdala-governed stress response—sham acupuncture does not stimulate these same biochemical changes in our brain. Similarly, while real acupuncture creates changes in the brain stem and interior areas associated with long-term symptom relief, sham acupuncture affects only areas of the brain associated with the temporary relief of pain. Clearly, the success of real acupuncture is due to a deeper biochemical and more sustained brain-modulating effect.

Sham acupuncture's temporary pain and symptom relief may stem in some part from the fact that it stimulates key pressure points in the body, despite there being no needle penetration. Stimulating key pressure points without needles is, after all, what acupressure, another long-standing Chinese healing approach, is based upon. Acupressure, we know, is a well-proven and effective treatment in difficult-to-treat conditions, including nausea. In other words, the surprising findings in sham acupuncture studies may simply be an indicator of acupressure's power to give some measure of temporary pain relief.

It seems the benefits of sham acupuncture are echoes—impressive echoes, but echoes all the same—of the real thing.

Yet the fact that these echoes are so tangible challenges us to look deeper and ask whether something else is going on in the practitioner-patient relationship when both types of acupuncture are practiced that might enhance our healing through additional pathways we don't yet completely comprehend.

Researchers hypothesize that sham acupuncture's mysterious placebo benefits might best be attributed to several factors: the practitioner's conviction that the treatment will work, which is conveyed to patients and reinforces their belief that acupuncture will help eradicate their symptoms; patients' enthusiasm for acupuncture treatment and their personal faith in its benefits based on what they've been told or heard; and the holistic way in which acupuncturists communicate with their patients, treating not just their symptoms, but taking a deeper interest in their entire life history, including devoting a significant amount of time in both the initial intake and subsequent visits to discussing an individual's childhood history and current lifestyle, and the pressing emotional and physical stressors that may influence his or her pain and health.

Their untold story is told. Words work their power.

During treatment, the acupuncturist also interacts with the patient in a physically attenuated way—holding the patient's hand gently as he or she studies the patient's pulse for a full minute or two, carefully placing each needle (or even sham needle), taking the pulse again after the needles come out and seeing what's changed.

These interpersonal interactions with a healing practitioner may in and of themselves be enough to stimulate or enhance the placebo effect to the extent that pain, anxiety, and other symptoms are, at least temporarily, blunted.

I think of something I recently read—almost humorous—that simply running your fingers over money relieves chronic pain. Having a practitioner place so much emotional and physical attention on you, your story, and well-being may be a bit like smoothing your hand over a million-dollar bill.

Indeed, MRIs of patients' brains show that real acupuncture does something quite extraordinary to the placebo effect itself: placement of needles in key meridians directly stimulates the area in our brain that governs our placebo response, or the expectation of a good, pain-free outcome.

Which is, in a sense, the icing on the cake. Real acupuncture alters key biological processes in the brain and, for added measure, increases our expectation that those shifts will evolve into lasting and profound changes in our bodies and in our health. That expectation, in turn, leads to healthier outcomes.

Rowland-Seymour has mentioned to me several times that acupuncture has helped a great many of her patients. That's why it was one of the first modalities she suggested when we began our doctor-patient journey toward the last best cure. She's seen what it does for her patients, just as my father-in-law once saw what it did for the patients on whom he operated.

I can't help but think back to a conversation I had recently with Trish Magyari as our *sangha* was finishing one night, in which I mentioned to her that I had recently started acupuncture. "That's wonderful," she said, smiling her inimitable smile. "I notice that when people who are practicing mindfulness also get acupuncture, their healing accelerates."

Moving Qi

Janet Althen is one of the few acupuncturists in the Baltimore area specifically trained to treat infertility; the wall full of new baby pictures in her Women's Acupuncture Center attests to her prolific success. But more frequently she helps women navigate the hormonal and physical shifts that come with exiting our childbearing years: moving from perimenopause into menopause. She has a philosophy, she says, that by healing women one by one she'll help each to become more influential and powerful in her family and community—and from there, more women's healing energy will help to heal the world.

It's a mission that began eighteen years ago when Janet was a single mom living on food stamps in public-assisted housing, managing a women's gym, and raising her young daughter paycheck to paycheck. She realized she needed more than just her high school degree to have the life she envisioned. She applied for grants to go back to school and get her college diploma. She started at a local community college and worked three part-time jobs to pay the bills until, five years later, she was closing in on finishing a four-year degree in communications. Still, she wasn't sure what she wanted to do.

The stress during those years was unfathomable: raising a young daughter single-handedly, three jobs, bills to pay, college papers due.

She began getting regular migraines that landed her in bed some days. She had no health insurance—she couldn't afford it. A close friend had recently recovered from severe kidney problems with the help of an acupuncturist; Janet decided to see the acupuncturist, too. She was hopeful, she says, that "I wouldn't just get treatment for my migraines. I'd prevent myself from getting sicker and needing health insurance, which I couldn't afford."

Acupuncture helped to keep the migraines at bay. A few months later she was getting close to graduation. Janet was lying on a treatment table and confessing to her acupuncturist that she wasn't sure what direction she wanted to go in terms of her career. Her acupuncturist asked her, "Well, what do you *want* to do?"

"No one had ever asked me that question before in my life," Janet tells me. "I was forty-two years old. I'd always done what I had to do, what I was expected to do, should do, could do, or what others thought I ought to do. I started to cry. What did I *want* to do? And the answer just came to me: 'I want to work from my heart to help women.'"

Cobbling together student loans and scholarship money—still working part-time, still raising her daughter alone—nine years later she graduated as a licensed acupuncturist. In 2001 she opened her practice, began to see patients, and finally began pulling in a regular income. From there it was an all-out effort to keep her practice up and running, and turn it into a success. Ironically, she was giving acupuncture to a dozen patients a day but was far too busy to take time to get the regular prophylactic treatments that had inspired her to study acupuncture in the first place.

Then, just as everything began to come together, her carefully stitched dream unraveled. At the end of her ten-year marathon Janet's body buckled under the effects of endless pedal-to-the-metal stress. She developed Hashimoto's, an autoimmune thyroid disease, as well as severe adrenal fatigue. "I had never been so tired in my life," she recalls. "My daughter, thankfully, had just left for college so she no longer needed me. I would go in, see patients, give them every bit of energy I had, and then come home and collapse on the couch."

Janet went on thyroid medication. She changed her diet. But she still felt as if she were, she says, dying. "I remember thinking, 'I'm never going to get better; I'm so tired I'll never get off my couch.' It was a very dark time."

An acupuncturist friend came to her apartment several times and tried a number of different treatments focusing on clearing past and present stress from the meridians of the body.

"That course of treatment helped me find my way back," she says. "First, it helped me to relax. I began to have a little more energy. That made me feel hopeful." Slowly, she says, "I turned a corner and got back on my feet."

"That experience really informed my practice," she says. "I had heard so many of my female patients complain of fatigue but I hadn't really understood what the word 'fatigue' meant until it laid me flat personally. Until I was the one who couldn't get off my couch."

Understanding what it feels like to be the patient while treating women has been, she says, as she touches the round turquoise and gold medallion that hangs from a chain on her neck, "quite extraordinary."

"In what way?" I ask.

"Many of the women who come into my practice have had their share of medical issues, immune and hormonal imbalances, pain, fatigue, life difficulties, and stresses," she explains. "When they come in I take an extensive life history. I've been struck over the years by the fact that quite often the women who come to me with such pain and fatigue have had very stressful lives. Often, they've had painful childhoods."

"As they go through treatments I see how acupuncture helps to move all that bottled-up stress and trauma out of their bodies," she goes on. "They begin to change both physically and emotionally."

This process occurs, she contends, for several reasons. Acupuncture, Althen believes, stimulates the meridians of the body to clear the emotional pain that our physical body holds onto when we experience childhood or adult stress and trauma. And, as this clearing takes place, as we lie on the table, still and silent, we also get to experience a sense of being right here, right now, our qi moving through us in a way we don't often get to feel. We experience the present in the same way we might in meditation.

Acupuncture, says Janet, "gives us the gift of sensing who we really are, a moment to reconnect to ourselves and our own energy." Once we have a regular experience of that, we begin to understand that it can be had. And that also helps us to make changes in our lives so that we make ourselves available to experience that feeling of well-being even more. "We become hungry for it," she explains.

But something else happens as we look through that quiet window into our own experience. "When we put down the mantle of stress that we carry every moment, we become keen observers of what those stresses are," Janet says. "I watch, over time, as the women I treat finally start to see the blocks and behaviors that have been holding them back. The grief they can't let go of, the patterns they've been repeating that are keeping them stuck." She holds her hands open on either side of her chest as if she's grabbing something immense that she wants me to see, hear, and feel. "Becoming that calmer, wiser observer unleashes something in them—their own healing qi. Their back pain gets better, their fatigue lifts, their hormonal imbalances balance out. Their physical symptoms subside. And at the same time, they feel a new energy—that allows them to become who they are meant to be." Her arms open wide, as if that something she wants me to see is huge, before she brings her hands quietly back to her desk, as if setting that something big down in front of me for my perusal. "Often, they finally start doing the things their heart has long been telling them to do and make real changes. They leave or start a new job or a relationship. Or they start a new career—like I did when I realized I wanted to devote my career to helping women heal."

IF I COULD, I would see Janet every other day. Because whenever I leave her office, I feel as if I've been meditating, only I've simply been lying still while she places needles in my head, my palms, my ankles, my toes, and unleashes my body's qi dance. If Janet could bottle the gliding-yet-grounded feeling she administers on her table, I'd stock up.

Meditation in a bottle.

But it's the physical shift I begin to notice that surprises me most. It occurs so naturally and gradually it isn't until after my fifth visit that I realize something is different . . . something big.

I leave Janet's office in my car. I fight my way through the beltway traffic. I stop by our new house to see whether the construction workers have begun pouring the foundation. I head on to our rented condo. I park the car and walk the dogs. Realizing that I need to conduct an interview in a few minutes, I race up the two flights of stairs to my office. I take the last few steps two at a time. A few seconds later I find myself standing over my computer, poised to pick up the phone.

What am I waiting for? I imagine I've forgotten some small detail— the phone number I'm calling? My prep interview notes? Then it hits me. My body is on pause. It is expecting that feeling: that knock-down-suck-out-your-bone-marrow fatigue to roll over me like a wave, causing my legs to collapse.

But the wave doesn't come.

I raced up the steps.

Nearly a year ago, when I started this quest, I'd come to accept the fact that hauling myself up the stairs and collapsing at the top was my norm. My body, like Pavlov's dogs, has been trained to equate flights of stairs with the fatigue that has defined my life. But little by little— with the help of meditation, mindfulness, yoga, and acupuncture— something big has happened: my norm has changed. My fatigue/ energy quotient used to be 90/10: 90 percent fatigue, 10 percent flickers of relief. If I were to calculate it now, my fatigue/energy quotient would be more like 35/65. When I have a bad day, it's how I used to feel most days. My good days are way more frequent—and better.

That's a gift I never expected to have.

I remember my neurologist once telling me, years go, that if other people with undamaged neuromuscular systems have a dollar of energy to spend a day, I have, by comparison, a dime. We can move around with just 10 percent of our nerve connections working in our legs, he explained. We can. But we are going to be mighty tired doing it day after day.

And that's why it's so shocking that, having raced through the morning as I have, my dime seems to be stretching so far.

THE NEXT WEEK when I see Janet again, I share my epiphany with her. And I add: "After I see you I feel like I have another layer of energy I've never felt before."

She's quiet for a second. "The question is, what is it you hope to do with this extra energy you're starting to have?"

I must look a little perplexed.

She smiles. "In Chinese medicine, the idea is that we only have a finite amount of life energy. Once we've spent it, that's it, it's gone. You've already spent more than most people do in a lifetime, fighting for your health, raising your family in between hospital stays, researching books, helping clients. Being constantly on, trying to put on a front that everything is fine—while fighting through a firewall of physical fatigue and pain." She taps the treatment table I'm lying on. "When you're here, we restore your qi. To you that restoration might feel like an additional layer of energy, because you've been depleted for so many years. But it's really just bringing you back to where you should be—into a balanced state of homeostasis. Your baseline. And that's a different thing. If you confuse restoration with 'extra energy,' you'll simply use that restored energy to deplete yourself more."

I think I understand. "You mean I'm finally approaching something close to a normal energy level, and if I use up that energy trying to accomplish even more in every given day, I'll simply defeat the purpose of healing in the first place?"

She nods, answering my question with a question. "What is it that you're hoping for in your life . . . if your energy is restored, if you're no longer held back by illness?"

"I've never had the luxury of asking myself *What do I want to do with all my energy?*" I laugh. "I've been in lifeboat survival mode."

"In Chinese medicine, perimenopause is a time when the blood rises upward from the womb and into the heart," Janet goes on. "It's a time for a woman to finally live from the heart, pursue what gives her joy, give to herself, rather than give so much of her nurturing energy to other people's needs." She pauses. "It's interesting that you're going through this healing journey at the same time that you're about to go through this next stage of your life. It's an opportunity to ask yourself not only how you might see yourself without illness, but how you see . . . you."

"I want to move on from the past," I say. "I mean really let it go." I pause. "And I want to learn to . . . relax and enjoy."

When you have been sick for a very long time, the word *relaxation* falls from your vocabulary. Instead of relaxing you rest and recuperate. You don't want to but you're forced to because getting done what other people do takes you twice as much effort and energy. And your body just gives out. Relaxation is something we do by choice. It's different from meditation or yoga or lying on an acupuncture treatment table working to free your mind of stress and worry and pain.

For me, it would mean letting go and having fun with life.

WHEN I FIRST came to her, Althen asked if I was open to being treated with a specific placement of needles thought to help clear childhood stress.

"Whenever you think the time is right," I said.

Now, after five weeks of traditional Chinese acupuncture, Janet thinks I'm ready for five elements, a type of acupuncture that she believes will help address my childhood trauma. Traditional Chinese acupuncture works by activating the qi through key meridians. Five elements acupuncture is rooted in the ancient Chinese philosophy that all life is based on five elemental energies—wood, fire, earth, metal, and water. These, in turn, relate to particular organs and emotions. The idea is that when our meridians are blocked in any one element, we experience physical and emotional symptoms in those corresponding areas. For example, when there is a blockage in the "element" of metal, there is less ability to heal emotionally from grief and loss, which causes havoc in the organs of the skin and lungs.

I prefer more Western explanations of how acupuncture might help us to heal. It's hard for me to sign on for the concept that tiny needles can touch childhood trauma. But I remind myself that although the metaphors used to describe ancient Chinese healing philosophy are unfamiliar to me, the precept that acupuncture can help modulate the pain and fear-reactive amygdala—which is programmed by our past experiences—makes perfect sense.

JANET SAYS SHE'D like to try a specific treatment that stimulates the key acupuncture points thought to have to do with moving through this old fear and trauma. I ask her to explain the exact process, but she demurs because she thinks I have a tendency to "overanalyze and overintellectualize what's happening" in my body. She wants me to "let go"—to "let happen what will." It's enough for me to know that the treatment she's going to administer is "a little like eradicating viruses in your computer's software." The treatment requires placing five needles along the center of my scalp.

I lie back on the crinkly paper that covers the patient table.

"You look like you have a blue Mohawk," she says, after a few minutes of carefully planting a row of blue plastic-tipped needles into my scalp.

I used to have a fear of needles, as many people do. But acupuncture needles are hair thin—a dozen can fit inside the bore of just one hypodermic needle—so most people don't find them painful. And they're absolutely imperceptible to someone like me who has been stuck with hundreds of hypodermic needles over the years for IVs and blood draws.

So why does my body suddenly jump a half inch on the table when the next needle goes in?

"Each of these needles corresponds to a specific point having to do with your childhood," she tells me. "You just jumped at age nine to twelve." The years when my father took ill and died.

As she picks up my arm to take my pulse my pacemaker goes off. This happens whenever Janet puts needles in my body. My heart starts beating so slowly that my pacemaker has to kick in to ensure my heart rate doesn't fall so low I pass out.

Janet leaves me in the room. I am oblivious to the needles she just stuck in me, even the last one. Within five minutes of lying down, I enter a deep state of *ommmm* without having to do any *ommmm*ing. My head feels deliciously warm. It's as if I don't have to reach for the breath. The breath comes to me.

I can feel the qi slowly begin to dance, as if the strings in the center of my atoms are shifting, utterly relaxing, my mu-opioid receptors binding, my adenosine enzymes rising.

I flicker in and out for a minute longer. My SI joint aches. And then it doesn't. And that's the last thinking thought I have. My thinking brain simply gets up and walks away.

Time passes. Who's counting? Not me.

Janet comes back into the darkened room. She doesn't speak. Nor do I. Speaking would be . . . distracting. I'd lose my place—like losing my spot in a book I can't stop reading and don't want to put down. I don't want to be spoken to or pulled out of the delicious world in which I'm floating.

I keep my eyes closed. I sense her standing quietly beside me.

"Are we doing okay?"

"Mmmmm," I murmur. I feel a little bit groggy. I go back to my twilight world.

HER HANDS, WARM and gentle, take my pulse one more time, in each of my wrists.

"Just let your mind relax," she says, so softly. "And let whatever happens happen." I hear the door open and click quietly shut as she leaves the treatment room.

My mind begins to drift in a way that reminds me of times I've been under light anesthesia. I'm . . . not here.

What happens is simple: I fall asleep.

HALF AN HOUR later, when I leave Janet's office, the state of floating relaxation stays with me. Even through the hectic dinner and home-work hour. Even when the printer jams repeatedly and ink explodes all over my hands while I am on the phone with Zen, who calls from the grocery store to tell me he can't find his wallet. I might almost describe myself as bemused. I order pizza.

My only worry, as I get into bed, is that having napped on Janet's table, I won't be able to fall asleep.

But I do. I fall into a deep sleep, without my usual tossing and turn-ing. This acupuncture thing, I am thinking to myself, is the way to go.

IT IS A few hours later, close to dawn, when I wake up, shaking, in a sweat. My heart is racing. All night—at least that's how it seems—I've been having the same dream. Over and over. A dream loop I can't stop.

I see it again, even as I sit up in bed, and stare at the dim shadows playing on the mirror over our bureau.

I am driving with my mother; it is a normal and nothing day. I am eleven or twelve. We are driving along our local two-lane highway. Someone is chattering on the radio about the weather.

And then we see it. My father's wood-paneled Ford station wagon on the side of the road. The side is bashed in.

My mother's voice is taut and high as she cries out, "That's your dad's car; we have to turn around; that's your dad's car!"

And we are doing a U-turn on the highway and heading north so that we can U-turn south again to get there. . . .

Then, in the dream that won't end, it all begins again. We are driving. Someone is talking on the radio. We see his station wagon; my mother cries out, "That's your dad's car!"

I try to shake myself from the dream's long arm, setting my hand down on Zen's back. I watch in the gray light as his body rises and falls with his breath. At first I think his back is wet—then I realize my palm is covered with sweat.

I know the dream is not a dream. It is a memory I lost, long ago.

I close my eyes. When I do, I am there again. It starts to happen once more. As it did that day.

I begin to cry.

I know why I can't stop seeing what I'm seeing. Dreaming what I've been dreaming. This one moment is the beginning of the end of everything.

It begins right there, on the side of a highway. And I can't stop it from happening, everything from unraveling. My future life disappearing in front of me.

This is the accident that causes my father's arthritic pain in his neck and his knees to become so unbearable that his doctor puts him on a long-term course of oral steroids. These are the steroids that his gastrointestinal surgeon neglects to take note of in his hospital chart, when he puts in sutures that are well-known to dissolve when steroids are present in the patient's system.

I am seeing—remembering—the day that seals my father's fate.

And in the dream I can't stop it. Just as I could not in real life.

The moment we are driving, my mother and I, right before we see the car, before she calls out—this is the last moment when I will ever feel safe.

I feel my tears drip the short distance between the corners of my eyes and the pillow. I get up and open the curtains. Pink light is streaming in across the trees.

I think of how each time a physical symptom of mine flares, the skull-pounding fear that rushes through me is as toxic and terrifying as the symptom itself. Every time Zen leaves the house I call out,

"Drive safe!" without ever thinking about why. Some part of me always has my heart in my chest, a little bit unable to let go of the fear of it all happening again. Being left behind. Leaving my children behind.

It doesn't have to be that way.

I have the breath. I have down dogs. I have eagle pose. I think of everything that surrounds me: my sleeping family, the friends I could call right now, at five in the morning, if need be. I have everything I need to lead a life more like the one I long to have. Dare I say I may even have the capacity to relax and be filled with joy?

A few nights later, I have to be at school for an evening event on college preparation. It's too soon to be in this moment in life, but we've arrived nonetheless. It helps with my stress quotient that I have just been to Janet's office. Three hours ago, I still had needles in my hands and feet and across my abdomen. My ordinary clutch-in-the-gut thoughts—*Christian is a junior*, and *How the hell are we going to pay for college anyway?* are muted. Thankfully so.

At school, I run into a number of people I haven't seen in months. "Do you have a tan?" one asks, incredulously. Another comments in passing, "Did you do something with your hair? You look great!"

This just does not happen to me. I am used to people saying things like, "Well, you *look* good . . ." The implication being . . . "for someone so sick." I've heard "You look good" as a consolation prize statement a thousand times in the past decade. I've never heard, "You look *great*."

An hour later an acquaintance comes up to me during a break and says, "Your face! You look . . . different! What are you doing? Can I have some?"

I am wearing a bright salmon color, instead of my usual black or white. So I point to my sweater and shrug. "It has to be the sweater," I laugh. I think for a minute of a good friend of mine saying once she could tell when I was having a bad day because I was "so pasty white."

Maybe I no longer look "pasty white" and people assume the change means I've gotten a tan.

"No," she says. "It's not just your sweater." She stands back, stirring cream into her coffee, looking me up and down, as if to take me in anew.

"It worries me," I joke, thinking of the stream of comments. "What exactly did I look like before?"

"Your face was kind of gray." She tilts her head. "And I know you were struggling with that rash. . . ." She is a dermatologist and we have compared notes on our distrust of eczema creams on the sidelines of kids' sporting events. "You were a little gray and white . . . and with the red scaling . . ." She flushes, her mouth gaping open, twice, like a fish, as if trying to recapture her words. "Well, I recall you were having a tough time last year. . . ."

I smile. I've always liked her directness. She knows I'm a science and health writer. I can take it.

She speeds up to get to the better part of her analysis. "Now you look pink! Tan!" She pauses. "*Different*. Really, what have you been doing? Tell."

The bell rings. Time to hear a timely if terrifying talk on college financial aid. No time to explain. "I'd have to write a book for that!" I laugh.

PART IV

Landing in
a Different Place

· 26 ·

The Final Reckoning

Anastasia Rowland-Seymour and I are ticking through our familiar checklist. Sitting across her ten-by-ten exam room on a black plastic chair is a young, second-year resident whom she's asked to sit in and observe. Like Rowland-Seymour, he's not wearing the requisite white coat. He learns fast.

"We were going over your file," Rowland-Seymour says. "There are a few things I haven't asked you about for a while." Her papers are out. All of them. "How are your headaches?"

For a moment I am baffled. "Do I get headaches?" I cock my head and ask this question with total seriousness. Then I remember. I was getting severe headaches with every menstrual cycle and we did talk about how painful they were—but somehow I've forgotten I ever had them. Or, maybe it's just that when I do get them, they don't have their old staying power. They last for half an hour, not two days.

Rowland-Seymour lets out a little laugh. "Good. And your irritable bowel? You haven't mentioned it for some time."

It doesn't take much to recall the gut-twisting pain I used to feel the first hour or two of every day. I remember worrying that I might not be able to handle morning yoga classes because of it. Then, slowly, the problem just went away.

"I'd forgotten all about it," I say. "I don't know if I could really describe myself as someone with irritable bowel. Maybe occasional touchy bowel syndrome."

Rowland-Seymour lets out another of her short, happy signature laughs. She flips through her notes. "I haven't written you any new referrals for physical therapy for your back, your bladder, or pelvic floor spasms, or your tendonitis for more than six months," she says. "Looking back at your history that's impressive. You've been in physical therapy for the past decade."

"Ninety percent of the time my back pain and pelvic pain isn't enough to enter my radar," I say. "I have to think about it to realize I still feel some twinging. When it's an issue I'm mindful of the pain and why it's happening and I adjust my posture. I do more yoga. More forward bends."

"Pelvic floor spasms?"

"Clearly the trick for pelvic floor spasms is to do lots of hatha yoga lunges and standing poses," I laugh.

"Has the yoga translated into the increased agility and endurance you were hoping to find?"

"I am not sure I will ever be able to describe myself as *agile*," I say. "But my core is getting to be . . . dependable. And building that strength makes me feel . . . ready for life in a way I never have before." I think of something else. "I haven't been wearing my hand and wrist braces for four or five months. I just haven't put them on."

"You would be if your tendonitis and inflammation were causing you the habitual pain they did a year ago."

I turn toward her resident. "I used to wear wrist and hand braces at night and when I was working on my computer. They're both in a drawer now." I smile and shrug again. "I can pick up heavier objects. Like large iron skillets. And I'm not dropping smaller objects quite as much. Things do still fly across the room—like my toothbrush this morning. But I hadn't dropped anything in so long it surprised me when it rolled across the floor." I rub my palms together as if to test my own words. Yes. I am better able to feel my own skin.

"What about your overall fatigue level?" We both know that for me this has been the big bugaboo. The joy thief.

"I sometimes get an echo of that old whoosh of fatigue. When I feel that first terrible sensation that my cells are all sliding south toward the floor I pay attention. I spend ten minutes meditating. Five minutes in sun salutations. See my acupuncturist. Write in my gratitude book. Walk outside. Stare at something small and startlingly beautiful. A leaf. A cloud. Send a deep layer of loving-kindness to someone who's driving me absolutely around the bend."

Rowland-Seymour and her resident exchange a glance. He slightly shakes his head as if to say, "I had no idea."

"And getting up the steps?" Dr. Rowland-Seymour asks. "That, I think, may tell us more than any of the lab work we're about to run. I'd go so far as to say it's your personal litmus test."

I relay how I recently went up two flights of steps, taking the last two steps at once. "I didn't realize what I was doing at first. It took me a minute to realize I'd raced up the steps and hadn't collapsed." I pause, worrying that in my excitement to relate how things have changed for me I might be painting a rosier picture than I intend. "Of course it isn't always like that," I caution. "Some days the stairs still seem evil. But that's the exception. And I can't think of when I last had to stop halfway up. Or lie down at the top."

Rowland-Seymour sits back in her chair, giving me that familiar, happy back-and-forth shake of her head, her dark brown curls, corralled by her ponytail, waving slowly in and out of view. "Incredible." She gets up, gesturing for me to stand up, too. "Let's see how your balance is."

I know the drill. The "drunk driver" test. How many times have I tried this, either in my neurologist's office, or here? And to no avail? I start across the tiled floor as Rowland-Seymour hovers a few feet to my left. One step. I place my left heel to my right toe as I start to take a second. And then . . . my right heel fits neatly against my left toe and I am . . . stable. Rowland-Seymour's hands are a few millimeters from my left arm, which I've stretched out along with my right in airplane mode. But I don't need her open, steady grip this time. There's no need to catch me. A half minute later I've crossed the entire, albeit small, room. I reach the wall and stand normally. "Wow," I say. Or maybe I say, "Whew."

Rowland-Seymour has the facial expression of someone whistling.

"That's incredible," her resident says, standing up.

Rowland-Seymour talks over her shoulder to him, her bright, warm eyes still on me. "She couldn't take two steps a year ago without losing her balance." She is visibly moved.

I feel, in that moment, like the rats that experience "spontaneous locomotion." "Watch this," I say. I am being a bit show-offish and obnoxious, but I am on a roll now, and I have so rarely been in a position to show off when it comes to my legs. I balance on one foot and go into tree pose, planting my right foot on my inner left thigh, slowly extending my arms overhead. I hold the pose, wobbling at first. Then, slowly, I center myself and move into the full expression of eagle pose, standing on one leg, my right leg wrapping around my left knee, my arms curling around themselves and rising in front of my face as I sink lower, holding in my core, holding. Muscle energy.

"You shouldn't be able to do that," Rowland-Seymour says, her arms rising, uncertainly, back up in the air to spot me. "*That* is not something I was ever expecting to see." When I don't fall, her palms turn up and her shoulders rise in what I recognize as her glad "wow" gesture. She breaks out laughing.

"If this isn't a testament to how we should rethink health care," Dr. Resident says. "I wish we could get every patient to do half of what you've been doing."

"I wish every patient had even half as good a doctor as I do," I say. "I hope you know you are learning from the best."

"I know," he says. "I know."

As we all sit back down, I nevertheless feel the need to follow my exhibition with a slightly more cautionary tale. "I don't want to overstate my case. It isn't that I don't still get fatigued, or ever have trouble with the stairs or feel my hands go numb. It's that my symptoms come less often, and when they do come, my baseline has changed. The starting place isn't quite so bad, and I come back to a place where things are tolerable so much more quickly. It's a bad afternoon instead of a bad month—or year."

"Your symptoms are quiescent," Rowland-Seymour says. "And when those symptoms flare you know what to do to help them return to that quiescent state."

I smile. "I like that word. *Quiescent.* Exactly. Things don't feel resolved, or as if they are gone; they feel as if they're not being provoked into agitated overactivity."

"There is something else really important," I add. "I used to have a symptom, and my worry over what it might mean would hit me like an almost physical second injury—that flood of cortisol, that negative floating brain coursing through me like a toxic injection. But now the ghosts of old memories of all the physical trauma I've ever known don't flood me with fear in the same way. I can ignore and even turn those ghosts away. Symptoms arise and I'm able to tell myself a new story."

"And how does that story go?"

"These symptoms are present now, but they will go away again. And, if they don't go away on their own, I can take action, call the appropriate doctor, go in for tests if need be—and yet still remain free in my mind to find beauty and joy and quiet as I do so." I think for a moment. "In turn, my symptoms don't seem to be as traumatic, perhaps because I don't *feel* as traumatized. It's not that my life or body are entirely different. I'm different in my body and in my life." I pause. "You could say my body is under new management."

"And do you feel going back to look at your childhood—your ACEs—has played a part in this change?" Rowland-Seymour says this gently, as if she's been waiting to get to this point in the conversation.

I sit back. "Yes. I have to say I wasn't prepared for how painful the process of meditating and being mindful and getting quiet to reflect on those connections would be."

Our visiting resident looks quizzical. He leans forward, his hands folded in a soft fist between his knees.

"It's as if, by getting quiet and going within, I discovered all these bandages that had been covering up a gaping wound I never knew was there," I say. "The kinds of wounds we all carry inside. I had to peel off that bandage." I search for the right words and they come. "After forty years I've aired out the wound and it's healed properly. The cellular pain of it is gone." I give a little head shake. "It's hard to believe I am sitting here still talking about my childhood—and I'm fifty-one years old."

Rowland-Seymour tilts her head, her brown eyes soft and thoughtful. "I have patients who are eighty-one and are still talking about their childhood," she says. "It's never too late, as long as you're willing to ask the question of what might be getting in the way of creating the joyful life you want to live now."

"Speaking of that," I say, rummaging in my workbag. "The joy test."

A YEAR AGO, Sanzone administered a test to me she developed known as the SJCQ-Inventory, or Sanzone Joy and Contentment Quotient Inventory, which captures one's daily perceptions of the world. Each question is answered on a scale of one to ten. I took my second SJCQ-Inventory last week. Rowland-Seymour spreads the two tests out side by side on her desk, comparing the results of the inventory I took a year ago with the new one.

The number 1 equals "Does not apply much at all/hardly describes my experience." A 10 equals "Nearly completely describes my perception/applies to me."

Here are my results:

1. "I feel deserving of a calm mind and a joyful life."

    A year ago I scored a 2. Now I scored a 10. There is no question, in my mind, that we all deserve and can have a calm mind and a joyful life.

2. "I am more self-critical and judgmental than I wish I were."

A year ago my score was a 9. This week I scored a 3. I'm never going to lose my inner voice of self-criticism. But I do know how to hit the mute button.

3. "I recognize and value unique contributions I bring to the world."

I was a 4 then. An 8 now. I doubt it sometimes, my ability to make a contribution to the world—but I have more faith that some small act of mine, whether it's smiling at a harried new mom in the grocery store, or writing about how to activate the healing areas of the brain, will help someone somewhere in some small way.

4. "In general, my negative feelings and thoughts impact my ability to fully engage with my life, including but not limited to people and situations or events."

An 8 then. A 4 now. I used to stew over pain and symptoms and painful people or what I did or said and I shouldn't have. I just don't do it as much now.

5. "I am more critical and judgmental of others than I wish I were."

A year ago I scored a 6. Now I score a 3. I still snipe at crazy drivers. I don't like it when the electric company forgets to put us on the electric grid. I get mad. But I hear my thoughts. I've become a cultivated self-observer. As such I have, I think, learned how to put a protective layer, a buffer, between what is happening and how I respond.

6. "Daily, I am touched or moved emotionally by things in my environment to a degree that reminds me of the goodness around me."

This was already high for me a year ago when I scored an 8. Now my score is a 10. There is not an hour that goes by that I'm not struck by something beautiful. The way water trembles in a glass. The way Christian is taller tonight than he was this morning. The glint of light through the prism of a pane. A neighbor smiling and raising her hand as she drives past. It's everywhere, every minute, the beauty of the natural world. The beauty of us.

7. "Generally speaking, my feelings or emotional states overwhelm me."

   I scored a 4 last year. This year, a 2. When my negative feelings overwhelm me, I execute an exit plan. If it's joy, I hold on.

8. "At least once a week, I allow myself to be spontaneous or playful without feeling guilty, despite my daily obligations and responsibilities."

   A year ago I scored quite high on this—a 6—solely because of my kids. If I were not their mom, and they were not so funny, I'm not so sure I would have scored above a 2 because so much of my adult playfulness has had to do with them. Or with Zen. Today, I score a 10. But it's a 10 that focuses on being playful in my own right.

9. "My feelings provide me information, but they do not control me or my decisions."

   I scored a 4 last year. An 8 today.

10. "In going about my daily routine I have difficulty being productive or completing necessary tasks without detaching from or shutting off my emotions."

    This is a big change. I scored an 8 before. Today, my ruminating or spinning thoughts get in the way of my getting things done about 2 percent of the time.

11. "I know specific things I want or need to change in my life, but I have a hard time putting forth sufficient effective effort to effectively implement them."

> A year ago I responded to this with a 5, because fatigue got in my way so much of the time. Now, my answer is a 1. Even when I don't feel like going out the door to yoga class, or meditating, I get up and go. And the rest of my day is easier because I do.

12. "I am open to new and different interpretations of my experiences."

> I was an 8 a year ago—now I'm a 10. This past year I've learned that my entire way of interpreting the world was based on a well-trained but flawed view. I've learned to deconstruct my experience and reconstruct it with a new worldview that's based on what's happening, right now, rather than on what's happening in my fear, my amygdala-fired-up imagination. I am open to interpreting the world through the Life Channel. I'm not saying I succeed, but I am open to it. And that opening is everything.

"AND WHAT IS Marla's take on all this?" Rowland-Seymour asks.

"She had a number of observations," I say. I relate what Marla has told me. That this year has allowed me to reclaim a sense of childhood optimism that seemed to be irrevocably lost. Which has opened me up to see the bright and color in the world, the good in people, in humanity and in myself. To be more playful, to "appreciate novelty," as she puts it, and to have a sense of hope and possibility in my future, even as I grow older. But perhaps most importantly, I tell Rowland-Seymour, Marla "believes that, whereas in the past emotional hurts and losses often became encapsulated in my body and manifested in illness and in pain," this has changed. As I'm experiencing less emotional inflammation, I am experiencing less physical inflammation as well.

"You've moved from fear to excitement about your life," Rowland-Seymour says.

I think for a moment. "Yes," I say. "Yes I have."

I DIVE INTO my workbag one last time and pull out the inflammation scale I filled out a year ago, as well as one I filled out just a few days earlier. The scale helps to evaluate one's degree of internal inflammation by asking two hundred questions about symptoms including gastrointestinal problems, neurological issues, headaches, muscle spasms and joint pain, fatigue and exhaustion, sleep disruption and insomnia, skin problems, and much more. A score of 0 to 10 is ideal. One hundred is considered severe.

"A year ago my score was 96," I remind Rowland-Seymour. "Now it's 33, about a third of what it was before." I pause. "Still way above the ideal. But I'm happy with that."

"It puts a number on what is an enormous and emerging change," Rowland-Seymour says. "I'm curious. How does the amount of time you used to spend seeing your neurologist, gastroenterologist, otolaryngologist, hematologist, dermatologist, cardiologist, urologist, pelvic floor specialist, or any of your physical therapists compare to the amount of time you spend practicing your current approaches?" she asks, mentally ticking them off on her fingers.

I do a little mental math. "For years I've spent three hours a week in physical therapy and another four or five hours a week driving to -ologists' offices in downtown Baltimore and waiting in clinic waiting rooms." I pause, checking my mental arithmetic. "That's about thirty-two-plus hours a month spent with medical care professionals—and that's when I've been stable; it's triple that when I've been in a flare."

"And now?" Rowland-Seymour is writing this down.

"Add up three hours a week doing yoga, half an hour a week practicing for ten minutes here and there at home, two-and-a-half hours in meditation every week either with my *sangha* or on my own, about one doctor's appointment every other month with you, which takes about an hour—and an hour a week seeing Janet. That's the same amount of time: thirty-two hours a month." I pause. "And those thirty-two hours are . . . fun."

Rowland-Seymour's intern laughs out loud.

"Have you compared it price wise?" Rowland-Seymour makes more notes.

I add up the dollars. "I used to spend roughly three hundred fifty dollars a month on copays to physical therapists and -ologists who have saved my life—and they've been worth every penny and more. Lab work and diagnostic tests have meant higher bills. A lot higher. And hospitalizations—that's a whole other stratosphere. But now my total health expenditure is close to half of what I used to spend on copays for physical therapy alone—about one hundred eighty dollars a month."

"So what have those thirty-two hours a month, or eight hours a week, taught you to remember when you feel exceptionally stressed? You're finishing writing a book and building a house that's been delayed several times. You're about to move. Again. And you have clients and their deadlines. And two teenagers."

"And a husband and two rescue dogs," I smile.

"And just a few chronic conditions," her resident smiles.

"That's . . . a lot," Rowland-Seymour says.

"My emergency toolbox consists of five very simple things," I jump in. I go over them all:

1. **Remember Why.** The science is real: your thoughts and state of mind direct your cells. Getting back onto the positive feedback loop isn't optional. It's your future outcome. I ask myself, Do I want to meet my grandchildren?

2. **Three a Day.** Use three of the myriad tools I've learned to activate the brain's healing response each day. It doesn't matter what they are or where I do them. Just that I do them.

3. **Claim a Quiet Space.** Take the time to go for a walk alone. Stare out the window. Be on the table at acupuncture. This hunger for

my own silent space is why we've taken a roomy closet in our new house and turned it into a yoga and meditation space that's just for me—something I would have felt terribly guilty about claiming for myself a year ago.

4. **Take Life Less Personally.** Remember that those around me are up against their own evolutionary biology, chemical reactivity, genes, and ACE scores. Recognize that in them as I recognize it in myself.

5. **Go to Class.** I am sometimes tempted not to go to class. To say I'll just practice on my own. But the truth is, I don't and won't do much on my own. And eventually, without the teacher support, my practice will peter out. And second, there is something that happens when we are with other women who are working to soften the same edges that we are. I do not know every detail of how this happens—the science on this is new and provocative. But the effect is real. Being next to people who are engaged in healing helps us to move forward, faster, too.

· 27 ·

Cells Tell

Anastasia Rowland-Seymour's number comes up on my caller ID: Johns Hopkins Medical Institutions.

"Hi!" I say. "It's the middle of the day. Does that mean it's good news?"

"I'm very pleased," she says.

All morning, I have been reading back through the early pages of this book. And here's what I've been thinking: I don't recognize the person I was when this journey began—the woman I see on the page. *Is that really me?* I have been thinking. *Was life that hard?*

And then the phone rang.

"Okay." I take in a breath. "Good." Conversations about blood tests always make me tense up and sweat, even now, when my doctor begins by saying she is pleased.

"Your overall white blood cell count is higher, which is excellent. Your lymphocyte count is higher. And your absolute neutrophil count is up. And that's all good."

"Is there a but?"

"No but. And."

"And?"

"Your complement factors are entirely normal for the first time."

I hear a note of excitement in her voice. "Remember, complement factors, C3 and C4, serve as the glue, helping our fighter white blood cells to adhere to abnormal proteins so they can destroy them. Your complement factors have risen significantly, which is what we want to see. That tells us that there is a marked decrease in your inflammatory response.

"Really?"

"Really."

"A normal range for C3 is 79 to 152. Yours used to be 70 or 75 every time we'd test you. Now it's 99. Beautiful. Your C4 has improved similarly."

"Wow."

"As I said, I'm very pleased," she says. "So, there is something else that's significant. Your red blood cell counts are now normal. And they're being produced at a normal size and at a normal rate. Your overall red blood cell count has gone up an entire point and since there is only a three-point range, a one-point change is rather notable." She pauses. "Your mononuclear number also decreased, which tells us that your long-term inflammatory process is less pronounced. It's still not in the normal range. But the improvement is there."

"The lovely take home here," she offers, "is that despite being in a highly stressful time of your life—moving, house building, raising teenagers, meeting multiple deadlines—you have built a resiliency that has allowed you to handle your day-to-day and have an entirely new quality of life both emotionally and physically. You might wobble, but you have the tools to be resilient in the face of what life brings your way. In every study we do, it all comes down to quality of life." She pauses for a minute. "I don't want you to get too attached to the blood work. Blood work is very changeable. You could have dips and swings in your blood cell counts in the future. But what matters is that you're able to handle your day-to-day life in a new way."

I sit with this for a minute. These changes give me hope that if one year of activating the healing responses of my brain can make a dent after forty-plus years of a negative floating brain, well, there is hope that in the next decade I can do even more good things for my cells.

I UNDERSTAND WHAT she is trying to say. I may have set out on a journey to find the last best cure, but in the end, I did not really find a "cure"; I found healing instead. Healing and being cured often overlap, but they are not the same thing. In order to heal we have to first embrace the truth that there are a range of emotional components that impact us at a cellular level in ways we still don't completely understand. And if we choose, we can make the effort to shift our state of mind away from pain and fear to joy and well-being, maximizing the healing responses in the brain in ways that affect our biology in lasting ways. Sometimes those efforts will result in a "cure" and sometimes they won't, but in all cases we will experience a sense of greater joy, of healing, that we can take with us throughout our lives, no matter what occurs.

Epilogue: Into the Wind

My birthday coincides with the full-throttle heat of summer and, often, our yearly vacation to the beach. Two days before our trip, Zen and the kids surprise me with a "comfort bike" as an early birthday present. It's made for people with shaky legs, poor balance, bad backs: the seat and pedals are extra wide and the bike, though light, is on a slightly larger frame to help keep the rider stable. I haven't had a bike in three decades and have accustomed myself, for years, to walking alongside my kids as they bike in the park or down the road.

I snap on my new helmet and take a slow ride around the parking lot that surrounds our condo. Claire rides beside me, watching every turn of my wheel. Zen is beaming at us both from the doorway, hands in his jeans pockets, Christian grinning beside him. Claire and I go quite slow at first. "Are you okay?" she asks, ahead of me now, her hair whipping back and forth as she turns to confirm that I am still upright.

"Do you like it?" She is sporting her Christmas-morning face.

"I love it!" I say. And then I just . . . take off.

"Mom!" Claire calls out, laughing. "Mom, wait up!"

And we are whizzing down the sidewalk, the green, happy leaves of the trees tapping me on the shoulder as if to say *go go go* as I zoom past, my daughter in pursuit of me, laughing. I switch into a higher and then higher gear. We get to the next big cross street and I come to a stop. She stops abruptly behind me.

"This is a seven-speed?" I ask, as we slowly cross.

"Yup."

"I need ten!" I say, as I peel off ahead of her, heading again toward the park near us, to a large paved path that meanders down a grassy hill through a stand of pines and oaks and ginkgos. "Seventh gear is too easy!" I call over my shoulder. "Slowpoke!"

I see the glee on her face. I cannot recall a time when Claire could look at me doing something remotely athletic or vigorous, without worrying over whether I'd get hurt.

Our bike ride has been on nearly flat surfaces so far. But as we hit a small incline my legs do their no-more-muscle-energy conk out, leaving me, momentarily, unable to turn the pedals at all. I stop. Claire flies past me.

"I'm just resting for a minute!" I call.

I need to pause but that doesn't mean I've hit flu-dog-fatigue status. I haven't. This is different. I'm exhilarated. My muscles are simply what they are. They need a little pause. Claire turns and rides around me in circles, waiting, smiling.

The reverberating eases. Thighs reengage. "Okay!" I say.

"Do this!" she calls out as she passes me. She throws her arms out to her sides, no hands. "Pedal one foot all the way down toward the ground and hold your legs really tight and still and you can keep your balance!" She has been thinking of this moment. Planning it. For some time.

I try it. I follow my daughter, spreading my arms wide, one pedal all the way down, legs locked, back straight. Whizzing past the pine trees and the green ginkgos and oaks. No hands! My hair is flying, I am flying, I am a bird, I am an airplane, I am five again, I am in love with this life.

Acknowledgments

Writing this book was a life-changing event. But transformation never happens in a void. When this project began, three women played an instrumental role in making my quest to find my own last best cure into the book you now hold in your hands. Dr. Anastasia Rowland-Seymour, my internist and assistant professor of medicine at Johns Hopkins, encouraged me to investigate how the science of joy might help me, and my readers, to heal. When I met the inevitable low points along the way, her inimitable warmth and humor, vast fund of knowledge, and stalwart encouragement gave me courage as we searched for answers together. In the process she modeled how every doctor can and should partner with her patients in the search for wellness. My agent and dear friend, Elizabeth Kaplan, was the first to recognize that my search for the last best cure *was* my next book. She read pages side by side with me, gave honest feedback, and was never more than a phone call away. I am not sure if I am luckier to have her as a friend or as an agent, but to have her as both is a double blessing.

Caroline Sutton at Hudson Street Press championed the idea for this book wholeheartedly from the start and edited the book with an intuitive intelligence. When the book detoured in ways we hadn't expected, her faith that the book would be better for it helped me have faith in my own writing process. I'm grateful to be in the hands of someone so gifted in her craft. This book is as much a product of the wisdom of these three women as it is my own—though any errors or mistakes are mine entirely.

Along the way, a number of practitioners gave generously of their time, far beyond what one might expect in the standard teacher-student or practitioner-patient relationship—and they did so long before knowing that our work together would end up in this book. I am grateful to Stan Andrzejewski, Deb Donofrio, and Linda Howard for their time and instruction. I'm especially indebted to Janet Althen, MAc, Lac, Dipl. Ac; Tara Brach, PhD; Julie Madill; Trish Magyari, MS, CGC, MS, LGPC; Marla Sanzone, PhD; and Mira Tessman, PhD, for teaching me that there is another way, and not giving up on me when I had to try, try, and try again.

Likewise, a number of scientists patiently welcomed my queries about their work. Kaiser Permanente researcher Vincent Felitti, MD; Rick Hanson, PhD, cofounder of the Wellspring Institute for Neuroscience and Contemplative Wisdom and author of *Buddha's Brain*; Tonya Jacobs, PhD, postdoctoral scholar at the Center for Mind and Brain at the University of California, Davis; Matthew D. Lieberman, PhD, professor of psychology at the University of California, Los Angeles; Christopher Lowry, PhD, in the Department of Integrative Physiology at the University of Colorado Boulder; Charles Raison, MD, associate professor of psychiatry at the University of Arizona and former clinical director of the Mind-Body Program at Emory University; Clifford Saron, PhD, associate research scientist at the Center for Mind and Brain at the University of California, Davis; and Srijan Sen, MD, PhD, assistant professor of psychiatry at the University of Michigan Medical School, were particularly helpful as I asked questions that no doubt seemed to them to have obvious answers.

A number of trusted friends read pages and commented. Lee Kravitz helped me to shape the idea from its inception and made wise suggestions about what to keep and what to let go. Jennifer Braunschweiger, my brilliant editor at *More* magazine, helped me cull pages early in the process. My dear friend Kimberly Minear acted as my first, brave "test reader." Jen Britton and Barbee Whitaker added important comments. My friend Peg McCarthy, PhD, professor and chair of the Department of Pharmacology at the University of Maryland School of Medicine, graciously added to my overall understanding of the science in significant ways, suggesting small but crucial changes.

Two dear friends offered places to write. Lois Lipsett opened up her home in Bethany Beach—"Grandma's Grotto"—to me on more than one occasion, saving me at junctures when I needed space and time to think and write and could find none. I will never forget her generosity, nor that of Minoo and Nader Tavakoli, who also gave me use of their beach hideaway.

During the time this book was written, we moved twice and built a budget-conscious house. Mark Giarraputo and John Clark, architects of Studio Z Design Concepts, kept me laughing through difficult house-building passages so I could focus on writing the passages of this book. My thanks.

Finally, to my husband, Zen, and to my children, Christian and Claire—in so many moments and in endless ways, the joy begins with you.

Appendix:
Finding Your Own Last Best Cure

Each person's journey toward the last best cure will be unique to his or her needs and circumstances. As you begin your own quest for a greater sense of emotional and physical well-being, ask yourself a few essential life questions. Looking to the years ahead, how do you want to live out the rest of your life? What state of mind would you like to be in as you go through each day? Do you feel a longing to start enjoying being right here, right now? And what steps—of the many you've read about in these pages—appeal to you most as you seek to shift from the Pain Channel to the Life Channel?

The exercises and steps that follow will help you to discover more about how your mind and body might have been impacted, if at all, by any childhood experiences (60 percent of us have an ACE score of 1, and 40 percent have a score of 2 or more); what your general mindset tends to be most of the time; and how to jump-start your own search for the last best cure.

1. Find Out If You Have an ACE Score.

The ACE score is a diagnostic tool developed by the ACE Study, a collaboration between the Centers for Disease Control and Prevention and Kaiser Permanente. Lead investigators Robert F. Anda, MD, MS, and Vincent J. Felitti, MD, have set out to help unveil the link between childhood adversity and adult health consequences.

They look at whether individuals experienced any of the following situations in their home prior to the age of eighteen: emotional or physical neglect; recurrent emotional or physical abuse; contact sexual abuse; living with someone in the home who is chronically depressed, mentally ill, institutionalized, or suicidal; living in a home in which there is an alcohol/and or drug abuser, or an incarcerated household member; living in a home where the mother in the home is treated violently; or having one or no parents.

What's My ACE Score?

PRIOR TO YOUR EIGHTEENTH BIRTHDAY:

1. Did a parent or other adult in the household **often or very often** . . . Swear at you, insult you, put you down, or humiliate you? **or** Act in a way that made you afraid that you might be physically hurt?

   Yes   No

   If yes, enter 1 _____

2. Did a parent or other adult in the household **often or very often** . . . Push, grab, slap, or throw something at you? **or Ever** hit you so hard that you had marks or were injured?

   Yes   No

   If yes, enter 1 _____

3. Did an adult or person at least five years older than you **ever** . . . Touch or fondle you or have you touch his or her body in a

sexual way? **or** Attempt or actually have oral, anal, or vaginal intercourse with you?

Yes   No

If yes, enter 1 _____

4. Did you **often or very often** feel that . . . No one in your family loved you or thought you were important or special? **or** Your family didn't look out for each other, feel close to each other, or support each other?

Yes   No

If yes, enter 1 _____

5. Did you **often or very often** feel that . . . You didn't have enough to eat, had to wear dirty clothes, and had no one to protect you? **or** Your parents were too drunk or high to take care of you or take you to the doctor if you needed it?

Yes   No

If yes, enter 1 _____

6. Was a biological parent **ever** lost to you through divorce, abandonment, or other reason?

Yes   No

If yes, enter 1 _____

7. Was your mother or stepmother: **Often or very often** pushed, grabbed, slapped, or had something thrown at her? **or Sometimes, often, or very often** kicked, bitten, hit with a fist, or hit with something hard? **Or Ever** repeatedly hit over at least a few minutes or threatened with a gun or knife?

Yes   No

If yes, enter 1 _____

8. Did you live with anyone who was a problem drinker or alcoholic, or who used street drugs?

Yes   No

If yes, enter 1 _____

9. Was a household member depressed or mentally ill, or did a household member attempt suicide?

Yes   No

If yes, enter 1 _____

10. Did a household member go to prison?

Yes   No

If yes, enter 1 _____

Now ADD UP your "Yes" answers: _____ This is your ACE score.

As we've seen, the higher one's ACE score, the more likely one is to experience illnesses including medical conditions and depression in adulthood. If you find you do have an ACE score, before going forward, consider talking through the results and how the past might be impacting you now with a trusted professional counselor or therapist. You can find out more about the Adverse Childhood Experience (ACE) Study at www.acestudy.org.

2. What Is Your Daily Joy and Contentment Quotient?

The following quiz will help you to gain insight into the way in which you relate to and react to the world around you, and how it reflects on your general state of contentment and capacity for joy. The joy quotient is an insightful gauge. In the course of my one-year journey my joy score doubled, taking me on Sanzone's scoring scale from "few moments of joy" and "a tendency toward pessimism" to a "considerably higher sense of contentment and fairly frequent experiences of joy."

*Sanzone Joy and Contentment Quotient–Inventory
(SJCQ-Inventory)*

Circle 1 to 10, according to the degree to which each statement applies to you or accurately describes your recent (past three months) perception(s).

1 = does not apply to me much at all/hardly describes my perception at all
10 = nearly completely describes my perception/applies to me

1. I feel deserving of a calm mind and a joyful life.

   1   2   3   4   5   6   7   8   9   10

2. I am more self-critical and judgmental than I wish I were.

   1   2   3   4   5   6   7   8   9   10

3. I recognize and value unique contributions I bring to the world.

   1   2   3   4   5   6   7   8   9   10

4. In general, my negative feelings and thoughts impact my ability to fully engage with my life, including but not limited to people and situations or events.

   1   2   3   4   5   6   7   8   9   10

5. I am more critical and judgmental of others than I wish I were.

   1   2   3   4   5   6   7   8   9   10

6. Daily, I am touched or moved emotionally by things in my environment to a degree that reminds me of the goodness around me.

    1   2   3   4   5   6   7   8   9   10

7. Generally speaking, my feelings or emotional states overwhelm me.

    1   2   3   4   5   6   7   8   9   10

8. At least once a week, I allow myself to be spontaneous and playful without feeling guilty, despite my daily obligations and responsibilities.

    1   2   3   4   5   6   7   8   9   10

9. My feelings provide me information, but they do not control me nor my decisions.

    1   2   3   4   5   6   7   8   9   10

10. In going about my daily routine I have difficulty being productive or completing necessary tasks without detaching from or shutting off my emotions.

    1   2   3   4   5   6   7   8   9   10

11. I know specific things I want or need to change in my life, but I have a hard time putting forth sufficient effective effort to effectively implement them.

    1   2   3   4   5   6   7   8   9   10

12. I am open to new and different interpretations of my experiences.

    1   2   3   4   5   6   7   8   9   10

SCORING:

For questions 1, 3, 6, 8, 9, 12: add up the exact numerical value of each answer you circled. For instance, if you circled a 4 for question 1, and a 7 for question 3, add 4 and 7 together and continue adding the number value of each answer for these questions.

Put your score here:_____

For questions 2, 4, 5, 7, 10, 11: add up your scores in the reverse direction. In other words, a 1 gets 10 points, whereas a 10 gets 1 point. A 2 would be an 8. A 4 would be a 7, and so on.

Put your score here: _____

Now, add up your two scores:_____

Less than 38 total points: Significantly less contentment and considerably fewer moments of joy than most report experiencing. Could benefit from concerted effort toward increasing both greater life satisfaction and feelings of well-being.

39–59 points: Occassional but not frequent sense of general contentment, and few moments of joy that you are likely not inclined to expect. Average or "middle-of-the-road" sense of life satisfaction and well-being. You may desire more experiences of joy and an increased sense of happiness, but may recognize a tendency toward pessimism and a general belief that you don't deserve or shouldn't expect more positive experiences than you have.

60–78 points: General sense of contentment and occassional moments of joy that you look forward to and work toward. Above average sense of life satisfaction and overall positive view of self and the world around you. You believe you deserve a satisfying life, generally are not overly pessimistic, and at times have a relatively optimistic but not idealistic worldview.

Above 79 points: Considerably higher sense of contentment and fairly frequent experiences of joy. Greater general life satisfaction and well-being than most. You tend toward optimism and at times even idealism, which you are likely to find refreshing and fun.

Copyright Marla Sanzone, PhD, 2013

If you find that your scores reflect less of a sense of overall contentment than you'd like to have, it can be a good idea to go over these results with a professional.

3. Set a Goal.

You don't have to do everything. My journey lasted a year—but really it continues each day of my life. The benefits of the practices I've begun expand into my life in ways that make being here, right now, richer, more meaningful, and just more fun. Every day I have to learn it all again—it's just a little easier than it was the day before to stay with the program. The important thing is not to feel overwhelmed. Start where you are. Ask yourself: How much can you do? What are your physical limitations? What can you afford? Here are a few suggestions for how to get going right now—regardless of any difficult circumstances you may face.

4. Find a Mindfulness Teacher Whose Style You Love.

Mindful breathing is a technique learned and relearned every day over a lifetime. It's hard, if not impossible, to pick up and stick with such a life-altering practice simply by reading about it on the page. We all need a voice to follow, a teacher to model for us how to catch and stop the insidious voice within—the voice of not okay-ness—to learn to name our emotions, and stop "drinking the poison" of our own ruminating thoughts.

To find an MBSR class near you visit the Center for Mindfulness in Medicine, Health Care and Society Web site run by the University of Massachusetts Medical School (that's where Jon Kabat-Zinn first developed and founded the mindfulness-based stress reduction program) at http://w3.umassmed.edu/MBSR/public/searchmember.aspx. Fill in the "Search MBSR Member in your area" form. Most MBSR classes cost around $400 to $500 for a six- or eight-week intensive program. Some teachers offer discounts and scholarships for those in special circumstances. You can also call your local hospital or community center to see what courses they offer. If you prefer a drop-in meditation class, check out schedules at local yoga and meditation centers. Try several to see what meditation teaching style appeals to you. Many are offered for free, or for a donation only. You'll know when the teaching voice you hear as you try to settle into mindful breathing feels clear, grounding, and nurturing.

If you're having trouble finding a class, or can't leave the house, consider starting with a set of CDs. (And even if you do take a class, stock up on downloads and CDs for those days when you don't have class.) MBSR courses often provide daily practice CDs with course materials. And most local libraries offer general meditation CDs. Best of all, some of the most powerful teachers, such as Tara Brach, make their guided meditations available to all for free via their Web sites— with donations welcome. (I listen to Tara Brach's podcasts whenever I take the dogs on a long power walk. Her teachings are astonishingly restful and awakening at the same time.)

Here are a few of my favorite mediation resources:

Tara Brach, PhD

To find out about Tara Brach's teaching schedule, free downloadable talks, and meditations, go to her Web site: www.tarabrach.com. Pick up her books *Radical Acceptance* (Bantam, 2003) and *True Refuge* (Bantam, 2013). And check out her blog at blog.tarabrach.com.

Trish Magyari, MS, CGC, MS, LGPC

Learn more about Trish Magyari's guided meditations, which are available on CD, at trishmagyari.com. You can also find out more about her mindfulness-based stress reduction (MBSR) courses, counseling services, retreats, and trainings.

Sharon Salzberg

One of the greatest meditation teachers of all time, Salzberg offers meditations for download at no cost, as well as CD offerings and books for purchase at her Web site. She also teaches at retreats nationwide. See www.sharonsalzberg.com.

Pema Chödrön

Chödrön's talks are available for purchase on CD or as audiobooks through her foundation's Web site, www.pemachodronfoundation.org. I am particularly fond of *True Happiness*.

John Makransky

Author and meditation teacher Makransky teaches a beautiful and moving meditation called "Identifying Benefactors and Receiving Love," which can be downloaded for free at his Web site, www.john makransky.org. This meditation practice involves recalling those people in your life who have made you feel particularly safe and loved—in whose presence you've felt deeply valued for who you are, such as a favorite aunt or teacher or grandparent. Makransky walks you through this guided imagery exercise in which your "benefactors" make you the focus of *their* compassion meditation. It has a powerful impact. Makransky's books and CDs are also available for purchase at his Web site.

5. Track Your Happiness.

Trackyourhappiness.org is a new scientific research project that "investigates what makes life worth living." If you have an iPhone, use the app to try and get a better sense of how often your mind is in the present, and how it feels when it is and when it isn't. Bear in mind this isn't a scientific gauge; just the knowledge that you're checking in at regular intervals can skew your perspective on how you feel—but it's nevertheless a way to gain eye-opening insight into how much of your time is spent ruminating rather than engaging in what you're actually doing right now.

6. Move Mindfully.

There are three things to bear in mind when finding a yoga class: what style is right—and safe—for you, what can you afford, and who you gravitate to as a teacher. In order to find the two teachers and classes I frequent, I tried seven. Julie and Mira were best for me. I discovered two other teachers whose classes were terrific, but the times and locations, and their vigorous paces, made the classes a difficult fit for my lifestyle and body. Keep looking until you find a teacher who inspires you to keep coming back, whether it's a gentle yoga class that uses props or a hot yoga class that leaves you feeling cleansed. If budget is key, as it often is for those of us with ongoing medical bills, most yoga studios offer very affordable community yoga classes at night (often at half price or less).

You can also download free yoga clips on YouTube or buy CDs—but they are rarely a substitute for a live class. When the poses are done incorrectly yoga can lead to injury—especially if you already suffer from a chronic physical condition. Still, if you have a lot of yoga experience, videos have their place. Now that I'm familiar with sun salutations, I sometimes supplement my practice with a favorite Shiva Rea salutation I found on YouTube whenever I need to get my mood back on track, and am hungering for a little yoga lift, but don't have time or can't get to class. It helps me to achieve what yoga teacher Julie Madill calls the "cessation of agitation"—the gift that comes with our yoga practice. Still, I wouldn't have dared to try lunging or down dogging alone before I'd been taught by a teacher who could make sure I could (1) do it and (2) do it safely.

Something else happens when we go to class. We begin to grow as a group. When we're learning new skills we fire up what are known as "mirror neurons"—a particular type of brain cell that observes and receives signals from those in near proximity to us and triggers similar reactions within us. It's why we are more likely to start crying—or laughing, or yawning, or tapping our foot (or eating more potato chips)—if a friend is crying or laughing or yawning or tapping his or her foot or eating junk food. Our mirror neurons fire up in response to what those around us are doing and prime us to unconsciously mimic what we see. When we watch and imitate a yoga instructor, or even another student who knows the yoga ropes better than we do, our brain receives the information faster than we can by watching a video. Women have more active mirror neurons than men do, helping us to better imitate instructors. (This gender difference may be part of the reason why women attend so many more group classes, in general, than men do.)

Write down the times for your regular yoga class on your calendar two and three months ahead of time. That way when something else comes up (and it will) that slot is already taken.

If you're interested in the yoga teachers who've taught me, here's how to find out more about them:

Julie Madill

You can learn more about Julie Madill's yoga classes at maryland yoga.com. She has a unique ability to mix a gentle approach with difficult moves in a safe setting.

Mira Tessman

For information on Mira Tessman's yoga classes as well as her meditation retreats and counseling services see wellspringhealingarts .org.

Stan Andrzejewski

Stan Andrzejewski is cofounder of Greater Baltimore Yoga in Baltimore, Maryland. You can learn more about his hatha yoga physical therapy services and yoga classes at marylandyoga.com.

Linda Howard

Iyengar yoga teacher Linda Howard, with whom I also briefly worked, helps ensure that even those facing severe physical challenges can do postures safely with the aid of belts, chairs, and blocks. I often use Linda's interactive DVD—it allows you to input your physical limitations and select a preferred routine. The DVD program then creates a tailor-made practice for you based on your personal limitations: www.easingintoyoga.com.

Baltimore Yoga Village

Sometimes I take drop-in classes here—the studio and teachers have a special warm charm: baltimoreyogavillage.com. Owner Anjali Sunita is a brilliant teacher of both yoga and yogic deep breathing.

7. Do a Breath Exercise Every Day.

The gateway to calming down the sympathetic nervous system and activating the parasympathetic nervous system in both meditation and yoga is the breath. Which means the breath *is* the cure. Bring in a specific breath practice every day—and come back to mindful breathing on and off throughout the day.

Here are the breath practices we've covered in these pages: basic three-part breath (p. 109), three mindful sighs (p. 109), Tsoknyi Rinpoche's rapid exhale exercise (p. 112), Andrew Weil's "relaxing breath" (p. 113), alternate nostril breathing (p. 112), ocean or ujjayi breath (p. 186), and Kapalabhati breath (p. 215).

It sometimes helps me to concentrate on a breath exercise if I place my right hand on my abdomen—and indeed neuroscientists have found that placing a hand on the belly while breathing adds to the calming effect.

There is one more active breath exercise called "breath of joy"—a sequence of four physical movements accompanied by four breath actions—which I've come to love. I practice this at odd times—it's a tool I've come to rely on when I need to activate my floating brain, fast:

Stand with your feet hip-width apart, and gently bend your knees.

First practice the four basic arm movements: arms out in front of you; arms out to the side in a T-like formation; arms up above you; and arms down to the side as you bend forward at the waist, sending your arms out behind you.

Practice the breath sequence: a three-part inhalation with one exhalation: in, in, in, out.

Now put it together. Each breath action corresponds to a movement of the arms:

1. Inhale through the nose and gently swing your arms up in front of you, parallel to the floor.
2. Continue the second part of your inhalation while swinging your arms open to the sides in a T-formation.
3. On the third part of your inhalation, swing your arms overhead, hands to the sky.
4. On the exhalation, swing your arms toward the ground letting your upper body fold forward, bending your knees, as you let out a loud "Ha!"

(For visuals, search "breath of joy" on YouTube—there are many examples that will be helpful.)

8. Take Note of What's Really Working.

Psychologist Martin Seligman, the director of the Positive Psychology Center at the University of Pennsylvania, has developed a technique to help us take in what's going right in our lives. The exercise is called the "three good things." I practice it every night. At the end of the evening, I think of three good, positive, happy things that happened during the day. I write them down. They might be as simple as remembering the feel of my daughter's head on my shoulder while we watched *Masterpiece Mystery*. Or seeing the first fall leaves flutter down impossibly red and gold in the afternoon sunlight. Or, it might be that for the first time I was able to succeed in a yoga pose I've been trying to do for weeks or months. Or I felt calm and at ease earlier in the day on the acupuncturist's table. It could be a small memory of feeling utterly content, or an event as major as finding out something wonderful has happened, like winning an award.

Then, per Seligman's instructions, I ask myself "why" each good thing occurred. It might be that I took the time to ask Claire if she wanted to snuggle and watch a show together, or made the effort to meditate outside after walking the dogs so I could drink in the leaves shimmering and dancing on the trees, or that I tried that same yoga pose a hundred times without ever giving up, or that I picked up the phone and made the acupuncture appointment despite my crazy schedule, or that I worked long, hard days with my butt in the chair writing the project that garnered a small award.

I take the exercise one step further. I put the large five-by-seven index card on which I've written my three blessings under my pillow. Sometimes I have trouble falling asleep, or wake up in the middle of the night, or too early. There are times when I have so much on my plate—more than can be done—that as I wake I feel my heart beating in my head as if the lining of my brain were the skin of a drum. My sympathetic nervous system is churning up the PIN response before I'm even fully conscious. I can't get back to sleep. But if I run my fingers over the now crumpled index card beneath my pillow on which I've written my three blessings, the lovely moments of the previous day come flooding back. I savor them again. It changes my heart rate. Literally. I can feel my pulse slow down.

Realizing why pleasant things happen in the first place makes me recognize and internalize what I need to do to make more feel-good moments happen tomorrow and the next day. And it does something else. Noticing what's working, what's going right, helps us to figure out what we love. The next day, and the day after, we gravitate to doing more of what yields that feeling of pleasure, because we are more keenly aware of what that is. We're on the lookout for the good moments that saturate us with joy and well-being—instead of being on alert for the next bad thing. It helps us to right the neurological imbalance that comes with the negativity bias we all have due to our evolutionary biology. We set in motion a positive feedback loop. We make the pathways in the brain that help us to gravitate to our positive experiences deeper, faster. We become a little bit more like Velcro for the good stuff.

9. Whatever You Do, Do It in Nature.

Nature nurtures, accelerating healing. Practice your mindful sighs while sitting outside in the backyard, or meditate from your beach chair as you sit beside the ocean. Do a little investigating. Find out more about the "nearby nature" parks nearest to you and take walks on their gentle hiking trails. Go for a walking meditation in the woods and drink in the sounds of nature. Forest bathe. Stare at the ribbons of light pouring down in a pine forest. Whatever beautiful natural vista is near you, go there. I've found a nearby nature sanctuary that offers a walking trail that winds back to a Japanese peace garden, a meditation bench in the woods, and a labyrinth. When I practice meditation, or walking meditation, in nature, I allow the positive effects that come with each to become more potent.

10. Remember the Rule of Three.

Pick three things from your toolkit to do every day. Go to yoga class, practice three mindful sighs at a traffic light, walk the dogs on a wooded path. Or do a morning meditation, practice breath of joy during a brain-fog moment in your workday, or do mountain pose while you wash the dishes. Fitting in the rule of three doesn't have to take up a lot of time—certainly no more than, say, going to physical therapy. Try to work your practices in wherever you are—at the grocery story, on the sidelines of your child's sports game. Be creative as you pull these practices into your life in small, but life-changing ways.

The point is this: to kick your parasympathetic nervous system and positive floating brain into gear, you have to get up and do something different. You can't just keep ruminating in the same old way and expect something new to happen. The strategies and tools are there for you to use; you just have to put them into action.

If you don't feel in the mood to practice a thing, try "inside-out practices." Smile until you feel like smiling. Laugh until your laughter become real. Science tells us that inside-out practices coax our mood along before we even realize our mindset is changing. Gradient, or faked, laughter leads to authentic laughing. Just holding a pencil between your teeth (which activates the smile response muscles) puts us in a more positive mood within moments; we think more happy thoughts. Don't wait until you feel like adding in practices. Add them in and see how it makes you feel more like doing them.

11. Retake the Joy Test.

After a period of six months, retake the joy test. Where are you now? How has the hard work of practicing these methods paid off in terms of feeling more joy and well-being as time went by? Have your efforts provided any palpable relief? What exercises do you want to make sure you keep practicing—in order to live the rest of your life meaningfully and with an enhanced sense of joy?

For more information and inspiration join me online at lastbest cure.com. I'll see you there—and we'll continue the journey together.

Notes

Introduction

xv   *I knew that 133 million other Americans:* Centers for Disease Control and Prevention: www.cdc.gov/chronicdisease/overview/index.htm (accessed March 20, 2012). See also Goldstein A. Study: 129 million have preexisting conditions. *Washington Post*, January 16, 2011; A1. These conditions include back pain and sciatica; irritable bowel syndrome and other digestive diseases; arthritis, osteoarthritis, and other rheumatologic disorders; chronic migraines; thyroid disease; multiple sclerosis, lupus, inflammatory bowel disease, type 1 diabetes, and nearly one hundred other autoimmune diseases; heart disease; depression, anxiety, and other mood disorders; cancer; fibromyalgia; Lyme disease; chronic fatigue syndrome; and chronic pain.

xv   *Experts predict that these numbers:* Chronic conditions: making the case of ongoing care: www.partnershipforsolutions.org/DMS/files/chronicbook2004.pdf, p. 8 (accessed March 20, 2012).

xv   *Women are more likely than men to suffer from:* Health, United States, 2009, with special feature on medical technology: www.cdc.gov/nchs/data/hus/hus09.pdf, p. 260, Table 53 (page 1 of 2; accessed March 20, 2012).

xv   *Ninety percent of fibromyalgia sufferers:* Resting brain activity associated with spontaneous fibromyalgia pain: www.eurekalert.org/pub_releases/2010-07/w-rba072910.php (accessed March 20, 2012).

xv   *We are twice as likely to suffer from depression:* Depression in women: Understanding the gender gap: www.mayoclinic.com/health/depression/MH00035 (accessed March 20, 2012).

xv   *individuals facing depression have higher levels of inflammatory chemicals:* Dinan TG. Inflammatory markers in depression. Curr Opin Psychiatry. 2009 Jan;22(1):32–6. Raison CL, Miller AH. Is depression an inflammatory disorder? Curr Psychiatry Rep. 2011 Dec;13(6):467–75. Haroon, E, Raison, CL, Miller, AH. Psychoneuroimmunology meets neuropsychopharmacology: Translational implications of the impact of inflammation on behavior. Neuropsychopharm. 2012 Jan; 37(1):137–62.

xv   *We are more likely to suffer more from irritable bowel disease:* Duenwald M. New remedies for a frustrating illness. But do they work? NYtimes.com, December 7, 2004: www.nytimes.com/2004/12/07/health/07cons.html (accessed March 22, 2012).

xv   *and arthritis:* This information comes from an interview with Jacquie Dozier of the Division of Adult and Community Health of the Centers for Disease Control and Prevention. We e-mailed on May 30, 2008, regarding statistics from the 2006 National Health Interview Survey regarding prevalence estimates of self-reported doctor-diagnosed arthritis by age and sex. In unadjusted analyses for 2003–2005, the prevalence of doctor-diagnosed arthritis among adults was estimated at 21.6 percent, or 46.4 million persons. Prevalence was higher among women (25.4%) compared with men (17.6%): www.cdc.gov/mmwr/preview/mmwrhtml/mm5540a2.htm (accessed March 24, 2012).

xv   *Women are three times more likely than men to suffer from:* See my book, *The Autoimmune Epidemic* (New York: Touchstone/Simon & Schuster, 2008).

xv   *Because breast cancer affects:* This statistic comes from an e-mail exchange with Busola Afolabi, media relations manager at the American Cancer Society, on May 28, 2008. Women have higher incidence rates of cancer than men in the younger age groups because breast cancer has a younger age distribution than most cancers.

xv   *We're far more likely to find ourselves facing multiple:* This statistic can be found in Johns Hopkins Medical Institution's publication, Chronic conditions: Making the case for ongoing care, September 2004 update. See www.partnershipforsolutions.org/DMS/files/chronicbook2004.pdf, p. 11, Figure 3, Women are more likely than men to have a chronic condition (accessed March 24, 2012).

xv   *both more emotional distress and a greater chance of disability:* Jennifer Kelly, PhD, presented these facts in a symposium "Translating Research in Women's Health and Mental Health to Practice," August 12, 2010, San Diego Convention Center, at a meeting of the American Psychological Association. She referenced the International Association for the Study of Pain's 2007–2008 report on pain in women: www.apa.org/news/press/releases/2010/08/gender-pain-differences.aspx (accessed March 26, 2012).

xvi *According to the Census Bureau:* invisibleillnessweek.com/media-toolkit/statistics/ (accessed May 18, 2012).

xviii *Even half of the muscle cells in our heart are regenerated:* This information is based on my e-mail conversation with Dr. Jonas Frisén of the Karolinska Institute in Stockholm, Sweden, whose work focuses on cellular regeneration, particularly as it pertains to the regeneration of the human heart. His work was recently featured in Wade N, Heart muscle renewed over lifetime, study finds. *New York Times*, April 2, 2009; A12: www.nytimes.com/2009/04/03/science/03heart.html (accessed February 26, 2012).

Chapter One

9   *Recently, I read a* New York Times *interview with:* Dreifus C. A nephrologist and patient. *New York Times*, November 29, 2010: www.nytimes.com/2010/11/30/science/30conversation.html (accessed March 22, 2012).

Chapter Three

17   *There is evidence, for instance, that if a mother suffers from a flu:* Kneeland RE and Fatemi SH. Viral Infection, inflammation and schizophrenia. Prog Neurospychopharmacol Biol Psychiatry 2012 Feb 10 (Epub ahead of print). www.ncbi.nlm.nih.gov/pubmed/22349576 (accessed May 23, 2012).

17   *Low consumption of fruits and vegetables in childhood:* Kaikkonen JE, Mikkila V, Magnussen CG, et al. Does childhood nutrition influence adult cardiovascular disease risk? Insights from the Young Finns Study. Ann Med 2012 Apr 12 (Epub ahead of print). www.ncbi.nlm.nih.gov/pubmed/22494087 (accessed May 23, 2012).

18   *Researchers were looking to find out whether patients had grown up:* The Adverse Childhood Experiences Study: www.acestudy.org (this Web site, accessed May 23, 2012 is currently under reconstruction, and as of this writing redirects you to www.cdc.gov/ace/index.htm).

19   *The average patient was fifty-seven years old:* Felitti VJ. The relationship of adverse childhood experiences to adult health: Turning gold into lead. Z Psychosom Med Psychother. 2002;48(4):359–69.

20   *But when the first study results were tallied:* Tough P. The poverty clinic. *New Yorker*. March 21, 2011; 25–32.

21   *He points me to a study:* Dube SR, Fairweather D, Pearson WS, et al. Cumulative childhood stress and autoimmune diseases in adults. Psychosom Med. 2009 Feb;71(2):243–50.

22   *In 2010, Felitti and his colleagues:* Felitti VJ, Anda RF. The relationship of adverse childhood experiences to adult health, well-being, social function, and health care, in *The effects of early life trauma on health and disease: The hidden epidemic*, ed. Lanius R, Vermetten E, Pain C. (Cambridge: Cambridge University Press, 2010), chap. 8.

22   *An ACE score of 6:* This statistic can be found in a transcript of a teleseminar session given by Vincent Felitti, MD, and Ruth Buczynski, PhD, "Why the Most Significant Factor in Predicting Chronic Disease May Be Childhood Trauma," for the National Institute for the Clinical Application of Behavioral Medicine, p. 11.

22   *Children who have a parent die, face emotional or physical abuse:* Dong M, Giles WH, Felitti VJ, et al. Insights into causal pathways for ischemic heart disease: Adverse Childhood Experiences Study. Circulation. 2004 Sep 28;110(13):1761–66. Brown DW, Anda RF, Felitti VJ, et al. Adverse childhood experiences are associated with the risk of lung cancer: A prospective cohort study. BMC Pub Health. 2010 Jan 19;10:20. Anda R, Tietjen G, Schulman E, et al. Adverse childhood experiences and frequent headaches in adults. Headache. 2010 Oct;50(9):1473–81. Goodwin RD, Stein MB. Association between childhood trauma and physical disorders among adults in the United States. Psychol Med. 2004 Apr;34(3):509–20. Dube SR, Fairweather D, Pearson WS, et al. Cumulative childhood stress and autoimmune diseases in adults. Psychosom Med. 2009 Feb;71(2):243–50. For more on the relationship between ACE scores see www.cdc.gov/ace/outcomes.htm (accessed March 25, 2012).

22   *Facing difficult circumstances:* Reeves WC. Childhood trauma and risk for chronic fatigue syndrome: Association with neuroendocrine dysfunction. Arch Gen Psychiatry. 2009 Jan;66(1):72–80.

22   *Kids who experience physical abuse:* Fuller-Thomson E, Bottoms J, Brennenstuhl S, et al. Is childhood physical abuse associated with peptic ulcer disease? Findings from a population-based study. J Interpers Violence. 2011 Nov;26(16):3225–47.

22   *Those who lose a parent in childhood:* Melhem NM, Walker M, Moritz G, et al. Antecedents and sequelae of sudden parental death in offspring and surviving caregivers. Arch Pediatr Adolesc Med. 2008 May;162(5):403–10. The children of parents who die suddenly are three times more likely to develop depression and are at higher risk for posttraumatic stress disorder (PTSD) than children who don't face such a difficult life event.

22   *children whose parents divorce:* "Is There a Link Between Parental Divorce During Childhood and Stroke in Adulthood? Findings from a Population-Based Survey," presented by Esme Fuller-Thomson, PhD, and coauthored by Angela D. Dalton and Rukshan Mehta, on Monday, November 22, 2010, at the 2010 Gerontological Society of America's (GSA) 63rd Annual Scientific Meeting in New Orleans, Louisiana. This paper is based on a representative community sample of over thirteen thousand people from the 2005 Canadian Community Health Survey.

27   *Research bears this out in myriad ways:* Cohen S, Janicki-Deverts D, Miller GE. Psychological stress and disease. JAMA. 2007 Oct 10;298(14):1685–87.
     The more stressful life experiences you face: Lantz PM, House JS, Mero RP, et al. Stress, life events, and socioeconomic disparities in health: Results from the Americans' Changing Lives Study. J Health Soc Behav. 2005 Sep;46(3):274–88.

27   *If you're stressed or depressed:* Searle A, Wetherell MA, Campbell R, et al. Do pa-

tients' beliefs about type 2 diabetes differ in accordance with complications: An investigation into diabetic foot ulceration and retinopathy. Int J Behav Med. 2008;15(3):173–79. Kiecolt-Glaser JK, Marucha PT, Malarkey WB, et al. Slowing of wound healing by psychological stress. Lancet. 1995 Nov 4;346(8984):1194–96.

27 *A fight with your spouse:* Kiecolt-Glaser JK, Loving TJ, Stowell JR, et al. Hostile marital interactions, proinflammatory cytokine production, and wound healing. Arch Gen Psych. 2005 Dec;62(12):1377–84. Gouin JP, Carter CS, Pournajafi-Nazarloo H, et al. Marital behavior, oxytocin, vasopressin, and wound healing. Psychoneuroend. 2010 Aug;35(7):1082–90.

28 *That's why individuals who regularly cite:* Davidson KW, Mostofsky E, Whang W. Don't worry, be happy: Positive affect and reduced 10-year incident coronary heart disease: The Canadian Nova Scotia Health Survey. Eur Heart J. 2010 May;31(9):1065–70.

Chapter Four

33 *In his book,* Full Catastrophe Living: Kabat-Zinn J. *Full catastrophe living: Using the wisdom of your body and mind to face stress, pain, and illness* (New York: Bantam Dell, 2009), p. 250.

34 *As Kabat-Zinn says:* Ibid., p. 255.

36 *This process of DNA methylation can occur much more easily within the brain:* My understanding of epigenetic changes in the brain was broadened by an e-mail exchange with Margaret McCarthy, PhD, professor and chair of the Department of Pharmacology at the University of Maryland School of Medicine, on March 31, 2012.

36 *These chemical markers disable:* I've based this description of Michael Meaney's gene methylation theory on that provided in the article by Paul Tough, The poverty clinic, *New Yorker,* March 21, 2011, pp. 25–30.

36 *Or, they might react in the opposite way:* Ibid.

36 *The good news, says Meaney:* Ibid.

37 *Researchers at Harvard:* National Scientific Council on the Developing Child. Early experiences can alter gene expression and affect long-term development. (Working Paper No. 10.), 2010: http://developingchild.harvard.edu/index.php/resources/reports_and_working_papers/working_papers/wp10/ (accessed March 23, 2012).

37 *This damage to the hippocampus:* Teicher MH, Anderson CM, Polcari A. Childhood maltreatment is associated with reduced volume in hippocampal subfields CA3, dentate gyrus and subiculum. Proc Natl Acad Sci U S A. 2012 Feb 28;109(9):E563–72.

38 *For instance, compared to people with no ACEs:* Dube SR, Fairweather D, Pearson WS, et al. Cumulative childhood stress and autoimmune diseases in adults. Psychosom Med. 2009 Feb;71(2):243–50.

38 *One of the physicians presenting:* Gretchen E. Tietjen, MD, director of University of Toledo Medical Center's Headache Treatment and Research Program, gave a talk entitled "Childhood Abuse and Migraine: Exploring the Relationship and Its Implications for Treatment" on Thursday, June 2, 2011, in Washington, DC, at the Annual Scientific Conference of the American Headache Society: www.eurekalert.org/pub_releases/2011-06/ma-caa053111.php (accessed March 25, 2012).

38 *Again, the ACE data:* Anda R, Tietjen G, Schulman E, et al. Adverse childhood experiences and frequent headaches in adults. American Headache. 2010 Oct;50(9):1473–81.

38 *And—perhaps unsurprisingly:* Chitkara DK, van Tilburg MA, Blois-Martin N, et al. Early life risk factors that contribute to irritable bowel syndrome in adults: A systematic review. Am J Gastroenterol. 2008 Mar;103(3):765–74. Heitkemper MM, Cain KC, Burr RL, et al. Is childhood abuse or neglect associated with symptom

reports and physiological measures in women with irritable bowel syndrome? Biol Res Nurs. 2010 Dec 30.

44 *A little perturbed by all that I've learned—and concerned that it might be too late:* McCarthy MM, Auger AP, Bale TL, et al. The epigenetics of sex differences in the brain. J Neurosci. 2009 Oct 14;29(41):12815-23. Nugent BM, McCarthy MM. Epigenetic underpinnings of developmental sex differences in the brain. Neuroendocrinology. 2011;93(3):150-8. Epub 2011 Mar 11.

Chapter Five

51 *I fill out an inflammation index with over two hundred questions:* The inflammation scale Anastasia Rowland-Seymour and I referred to came from licensed nutritionist Kasia Kines, MS, MA, CN, CNS, LDN, founder of Holistic Nutrition Naturally. You can read about her at kasiakines.com.

Chapter Six

63 *In one study, 72 percent of MBSR:* Kabat-Zinn, J. *Full catastrophe living: Using the wisdom of your body and mind to face stress, pain and illness* (New York: Bantam Dell, 2009), p. 288.
64 *One 2007 study Magyari coauthored:* Pradhan EK, Baumgarten M, Langenberg P, et al. Effect of mindfulness-based stress reduction in rheumatoid arthritis patients. Arthritis Rheum. 2007 Oct 15;57(7):1134–42.
65 *Yet after eight weeks the average participant:* Kimbrough E, Magyari T, Langenberg P, et al. Mindfulness intervention for child abuse survivors. J Clin Psychol. 2010 Jan;66(1):17–33.

Chapter Seven

67 *These researchers go so far as to say that:* http://news.harvard.edu/gazette/story/2010/11/wandering-mind-not-a-happy-mind/ (accessed March 25, 2012).
68 *it's what we ruminate over as we shower, drive, and fall asleep:* Hanson R, Mendius R. *Buddha's brain: The practical neuroscience of happiness, love & wisdom* (Oakland, CA: New Harbinger Publications, 2009). To hear a fascinating talk given by Hanson at Google in June 2010 see www.youtube.com/watch?v=0EM45CpeQb4 (accessed March 25, 2012).
68 *"If you drink much from a bottle marked 'poison':* This teaching can be heard on Pema Chodron's recorded talk, *True Happiness,* available on CD.
70 *The length of our telomeres is thought to be:* Kim S, Bi X, Czarny-Ratajczak M, Dai J. Telomere maintenance genes SIRT1 and XRCC6 impact age-related decline in telomere length but only SIRT1 is associated with human longevity. Biogerontology. 2011 Oct 5.
71 *Not surprisingly, they die younger:* Marchant J. How meditation might ward off the affects of ageing. *Observer,* 2011 Apr 23: www.guardian.co.uk/lifeandstyle/2011/apr/24/meditation-ageing-shamatha-project (accessed March 25, 2012).
71 *leading to pronounced and accelerated aging:* Tyrka AR, Price LH, Kao HT, et al. Childhood maltreatment and telomere shortening: Preliminary support for an effect of early stress on cellular aging. Biol Psych. 2010 Mar 15;67(6):531–34.
71 *This is related to women's higher rates of depression:* Figueiredo HF, Ulrich-Lai YM, Choi DC, et al. Estrogen potentiates adrenocortical responses to stress in female rats. Am J Physiol Endocrinol Metab. 2007 Apr;292(4):E1173–82.

71 *such as exercise:* Krauss J, Farzaneh-Far R, Puterman E, et al. Physical fitness and telomere length in patients with coronary heart disease: Findings from the Heart and Soul Study. PLoS One. 2011;6(11):e26983.

71 *and diet:* Farzaneh-Far R, Lin J, Epel ES, et al. Association of marine omega-3 fatty acid levels with telomeric aging in patients with coronary heart disease. JAMA. 2010 Jan 20;303(3):250–57.

72 *Surprisingly, some moms of disabled or autistic children:* Epel ES, Blackburn EH, Lin J, et al. Accelerated telomere shortening in response to life stress. Proc Natl Acad Sci U S A. 2004 Dec 7;101(49):17312–15.

72 *At the end of the three-month meditation retreat:* Jacobs TL, Epel ES, Lin J, Blackburn EH. Intensive meditation training, immune cell telomerase activity, and psychological mediators. Psychoneuro. 2011 Jun;36(5):664–81.

73 *It may even be that meditation triggers:* Epel E, Daubenmier J, Moskowitz JT, et al. Can meditation slow rate of cellular aging? Cognitive stress, mindfulness, and telomeres. Longevity, regeneration, and optimal health. Ann. N.Y. Acad Sci. 2009;1172:34–53.

74 *Aging, arteriosclerosis, and even recent viral infections:* Hesselink, J. Demyelinating diseases of the brain. This article was compiled by Dr. Hesselink of the Department of Neuroradiology at the University of California, San Diego, Department of Radiology: http://spinwarp.ucsd.edu/NeuroWeb/Text/br-840.htm (accessed March 23, 2012).

74 *Chronic migraines also damage white matter:* Kruit MC, van Buchem MA, Launer LJ, et al. Migraine is associated with an increased risk of deep white matter lesions, subclinical posterior circulation infarcts and brain iron accumulation: The population-based MRI CAMERA Study. Cephalalgia. 2010 Feb;30(2):129–36. Intiso D, Di Rienzo F, Rinaldi G, et al. Brain MRI white matter lesions in migraine patients: Is there a relationship with antiphospholipid antibodies and coagulation parameters? Eur J Neurol. 2006 Dec;13(12):1364–69.

74 *just six hours of meditation training and eleven hours of practice:* Tang YY, Lu Q, Geng X, et al. Short-term meditation induces white matter changes in the anterior cingulate. Proc Natl Acad Sci U S A. 2010 Aug 31;107(35):15649–52. In this study, scientists investigated a type of mindfulness training popular in China, known as integrative body-mind training, or IBMT. Quite similar to MBSR, IBMT involves focusing on the breath, catching habits of mind, use of mental imagery, and background music.

75 *Students who take a ten-minute lesson in mindfulness meditation:* Lehrer J. Under pressure: The search for a stress vaccine. *Wired,* July 28, 2010: www.wired.com/magazine/2010/07/ff_stress_cure/all/1 (accessed March 23, 2012). In this article Lehrer reports on a 2010 study led by Sian Beilock, a psychologist at the University of Chicago, who found that a ten-minute lesson in mindfulness meditation seemed to reduce stress in those taking a high-stakes math exam, leading to a five-point increase on average.

75 *Individuals trained in meditation perform significantly better:* Prakash R, Dubey I, Abhishek P, et al. Long-term Vihangam Yoga meditation and scores on tests of attention. Percept Mot Skills. 2010 Jun;110(3 Pt 2):1139–48.

75 *Adolescent boys who take four forty-minute classes:* Huppert F, Johnson D. A controlled trial of mindfulness training in schools: The importance of practice for an impact on well-being. J Positive Psych. 2010;5(4):264–74. See more at: http://mindfulnessinschools.org (accessed March 23, 2012).

75 *Remember earlier findings that those with ACEs:* Teicher MH, Anderson CM, Polcari A. Childhood maltreatment is associated with reduced volume in the hippocampal

subfields CA3, dentate gyrus, and subiculum. Proc Natl Acad Sci U S A. 2012 Feb 28;109(9):E563–72.

75   *Well, meditation, and mindfulness lead to increases:* Hölzel BK, Carmody J, Vangel M, et al. Mindfulness practice leads to increases in regional brain gray matter density. Psychiatry Res. 2011 Jan 30;191(1):36–43.

Chapter Eight

93   *In fact, the more mindful participants were in labeling:* Creswell JD, Way BM, Eisenberger NI, Lieberman MD. Neural correlates of dispositional mindfulness during affect labeling. Psychosom Med. 2007 Jul–Aug;69(6):560–65. Lieberman MD et al. Subjective responses to emotional stimuli during labeling, reappraisal, and distraction. Emotion. 2011 Jun;11(3):468–80.

93   *that patients who undergo talk therapy show brain pattern changes:* Miskovic V, Moscovitch DA, Santesso DL, et al. Changes in EEG cross-frequency coupling during cognitive behavioral therapy for social anxiety disorder. Psychol Sci. 2011 Apr;22(4):507–16.

93   *than the traditional treatment, light therapy, alone:* Rohan KJ, Roecklein KA, Lacy TJ, et al. Winter depression recurrence one year after cognitive-behavioral therapy, light therapy, or combination treatment. Behav Ther. 2009 Sep;40(3):225–38.

Chapter Ten

101   *Hanson writes and talks extensively about the complexity:* Hanson R, Mendius R. *Buddha's brain: The practical neuroscience of happiness, love & wisdom* (Oakland, CA: New Harbinger Publications, 2009).

102 *All our thinking, worries, and hopes:* Ibid.

105 *Everything we think and feel:* LeDoux J. The self: Clues from the brain. Ann N Y Acad Sci. 2003 Oct;1001:295–304.

106 *"that thinks it's always Threat Level Orange":* This comes from an e-mail exchange with the author, Rick Hanson, dated January 17, 2012.

106 *"DNA that down regulates the stress response":* Hanson R, Mendius R. *Buddha's brain.*

Chapter Eleven

109 *She sometimes jokes to her students:* The Venerable Khandro Rinpoche tells this story during a recorded talk she gave at the Mind and Life Summer Research Institute in June 2010 at the Garrison Institute, Garrison, New York, June 14–20, 2010.

110 *"And we build up tracks in our brain:* Trish Magyari drew this fact from *Concentration and Meditation*, by Swami Sivananda, p. 9, first published in 1975. Swami Sivananda cites his source as an ancient sacred yogic text, *Kurma Purana.*

112 *Cliff Saron recently sent me a talk that Tsoknyi Rinpoche:* Tsoknyi Rinpoche gave this talk at the Mind and Life Summer Research Institute in June 2010 at the Garrison Institute, Garrison, New York, June 14–20, 2010.

Chapter Twelve

115 *The Buddha taught them this practice:* This story appears in many places in Buddhist teachings and can be seen in full form here: www.urbandharma.org/udharma/metta.html (accessed March 23, 2012).

119 *Feelings of love for another activate the reward:* Younger J, Aron A, Parke S, et al. Viewing pictures of a romantic partner reduces experimental pain: Involvement of neural reward systems. PLoS One. 2010 Oct 13;5(10):e13309.

119 *A study following nearly four thousand:* Eaker ED, Sullivan LM, Kelly-Hayes M, et al. Anger and hostility predict the development of atrial fibrillation in men in the Framingham Offspring Study. Circulation. 2004 Mar 16;109(10):1267–71.

119 *And this correlation between feeling anxious:* Eaker ED, Sullivan LM, Kelly-Hayes M, et al. Tension and anxiety and the prediction of the 10-year incidence of coronary heart disease, atrial fibrillation, and total mortality: The Framingham Offspring Study. Psychosom Med. 2005 Sep–Oct;67(5):692–96.

125 *He confesses in his teachings that even he knows:* Tsoknyi Rinpoche gave this talk at the Mind and Life Summer Research Institute in June 2010 at the Garrison Institute, Garrison, New York, June 14–20, 2010.

Chapter Thirteen

129 *Or P over N (mathematically, P/N):* Fredrickson B. *Positivity: Groundbreaking research reveals how to embrace the hidden strength of positive emotions, overcome negativity, and thrive.* (New York: Crown Publishers, 2009), p. 16.

130 *Some studies suggest positive emotions:* Ong AD. Pathways linking positive emotion and health in later life. Cur Dir Psychol Sci. 2010;19(6):358.

130 *Of the sixteen most optimistic men, only five died:* Martin E. P. Seligman wrote about this experiment in his e-mail article "A Positive Psychology Update from Dr. Martin E. P. Seligman": http://app.simplycast.com/email_view.php?group_idno=5778484&outgoing_idno=5842970&email_idno=186643 (accessed July 31, 2011).

130 *In another cardiovascular disease study, which tracked over thirteen hundred veteran:* Ibid.

131 *As one famous study by Harvard psychologist George Vaillant:* Ibid.

132 *Which may be, they point out with all seriousness:* Nadler RT, Rabi R, Minda JP. Better mood and better performance: Learning rule-described categories is enhanced by positive mood. Psychol Sci. 2010 Dec 1;21(12):1770–76.

133 *Walking through a forest pumps up:* Lee J, Park BJ, Tsunetsugu Y, et al. Effect of forest bathing on physiological and psychological responses in young Japanese male subjects. Public Health. 2011 Feb;125(2):93–100.

134 *We even do better on memory and attention tests:* Maller C, Townsend M, Pryor A, et al. Healthy nature healthy people: "Contact with nature" as an upstream health promotion intervention for populations. Health Promot Int. 2006 March 21;(1):45–54.

134 *Patients with a view of nature and trees:* Ulrich RS. View through a window may influence recovery from surgery. Science. 1984 Apr 27;224(4647):420–21.

134 *When we seek out what researchers call "nearby nature":* Kaplan R, Kaplan S. *The experience of nature: A psychological perspective.* (New York: Cambridge University Press, 1989). Maller, C. Healthy nature healthy people.

136 *The average hug lasts:* Grewen KM, Anderson BJ, Girdler SS, et al. Warm partner contact is related to lower cardiovascular reactivity. Behav Med. 2003 Fall;29(3):123–30.

136 *They increase levels of the bonding hormone:* Grewen KM, Girdler SS, Amico J, et al. Effects of partner support on resting oxytocin, cortisol, norepinephrine, and blood pressure before and after warm partner contact. Psychosom Med. 2005 Jul–

Aug;67(4):531-8. Gordon I, Zagoory-Sharon O, Leckman JF, et al. Oxytocin, cortisol, and triadic family interactions. Physiol Behav. 2010 Dec 2;101(5):679–84.

136 *Just a soft touch sends a shot of oxytocin:* Kosfeld M, Heinrichs M, Zak PJ, et al. Oxytocin increases trust in humans. Nature. 2005 Jun 2;435(7042):673–76.

136 *Women who get more hugs from their husbands:* Light KC, Grewen KM, Amico JA. More frequent partner hugs and higher oxytocin levels are linked to lower blood pressure and heart rate in premenopausal women. Biol Psychol. 2005 Apr;69(1):5–21.

Chapter Fifteen

147 *In the past decade researchers have come to understand:* Tobin DJ. Biochemistry of human skin—our brain on the outside. Chem Soc Rev. 2006 Jan;35(1):52–67.

147 *Psychological stress worsens symptoms:* Oh SH, Bae BG, Park CO, et al. Association of stress with symptoms of atopic dermatitis. Acta Derm Venereol. 2010 Nov;90(6):582–88.

148 *This protein triggers a series of chemical events:* Attwood BK, Bourgognon JM, Patel S, et al. Neuropsin cleaves EphB2 in the amygdala to control anxiety. Nature. 2011 May 19;473(7347):372–75.

148 *However, the expression pattern of neuropsin:* Kuwae K, Matsumoto-Miyai K, Yoshida S, et al. Epidermal expression of serine protease, neuropsin (KLK8) in normal and pathological skin samples. Mol Pathol. 2002 Aug;55(4):235–41.

148 *Other significant studies on a brain-skin link:* Persson ML, Johansson J, Vumma R, et al. Aberrant amino acid transport in fibroblasts from patients with bipolar disorder. Neurosci Lett. 2009 Jun 19;457(1):49–52. Those interested in this topic might also be interested in this paper, demonstrating that skin conductance, a measure of the amount of sweating, can predict diagnosis with major depression with about 95 percent accuracy: Ward NG, Doerr HO. Skin conductance. A potentially sensitive and specific marker for depression. J Nerv Ment Dis. 1986 Sep;174(9):553–59.

149 *Lowry's work focuses on the relationships:* Hale MW, Dady KF, Evans AK, et al. Evidence for in vivo thermosensitivity of serotonergic neurons in the rat dorsal raphe nucleus and raphe pallidus nucleus implicated in thermoregulatory cooling. Exp Neurol. 2010;227:264–78. Kelly KJ, Donner NC, Hale MW, et al. Swim stress activates serotonergic and nonserotonergic neurons in specific subdivisions of the rat dorsal raphe nucleus in a temperature-dependent manner. Neuroscience. 2011;197:251–68.

149 *His recent paper, which has the entertaining title:* Lowry CA, Lightman SL, Nutt DJ, et al. That warm fuzzy feeling: Brain serotonergic neurons and the regulation of emotion. J Psychopharmacol. 2009;23:392–400.

151 *researchers at Cornell University:* Pattwell SS, Bath KG, Casey BJ, et al. Selective early-acquired fear memories undergo temporary suppression during adolescence. Proc Natl Acad Sci U S A. 2011 Jan 18;108(3):1182–87.

Chapter Sixteen

155 *That death "means nothing":* www.alberteinsteinsite.com/quotes/einsteinquotes.html (accessed March 26, 2012).

Chapter Eighteen

172 *This serotonin gene comes in three different:* Gene variants are also known as gene alleles. The term *allele*—which comes from the word *allelomorph,* meaning "other form"—refers to the different forms any one gene can take. For instance, our gene alleles usually code for our red blood cells to have a round, concave shape. But if there is a mutation in that gene, which causes another allele to be expressed, a red blood cell might be shaped, instead, in the form of a sickle-causing sickle cell anemia.

172 *A few days earlier I had a conversation with Srijan Sen, MD, PhD:* In this study, Srijan Sen, MD, PhD, assistant professor of psychiatry at the University of Michigan Medical School, and his colleagues examined fifty-four studies done between 2001 and 2010 looking at 41,000 individuals—the largest analysis ever done of the relationship between individuals' serotonin genetic make-up and how well they were able to bounce back from adversity. Karg K, Burmeister M, Shedden K, et al. The serotonin transporter promoter variant (5-HTTLPR), stress, and depression meta-analysis revisited: Evidence of genetic moderation. Arch Gen Psych. 2011 May;68(5).144–54.

173 *In individuals with the short-short gene variant:* Hariri AR, Mattay VS, Tessitore A, et al. Serotonin transporter genetic variation and the response of the human amygdala. Science. 2002 Jul 19;297(5580):400–403.

173 *We already know that children with a history of ACEs:* Aguilera M, Arias B, Wichers M, et al. Early adversity and 5-HTT/BDNF genes: New evidence of gene-environment interactions on depressive symptoms in a general population. Psychol Med. 2009 Sep;39(9):1425–32.

174 *We might extrapolate these depression findings:* Copeland WE, Shanahan L, Worthman C, et al. Cumulative depression episodes predict later C-reactive protein levels: A prospective analysis. Biol Psych, 2012 Jan 1;71(1):15–21.

174 *Having a particularly plastic brain also means:* Belsky J, Pluess M. Beyond diathesis stress: Differential susceptibility to environmental influences. Psychol Bulletin. 2009;135(6):885–908. Belsky J. Variation in susceptibility to rearing influences: An evolutionary argument. Psychol Inquiry. 1997;8:182–86. Belsky J. Theory testing, effect-size evaluation, and differential susceptibility to rearing influence: The case of mothering and attachment. Child Devel. 1997;68(4):598–600. Belsky J. Differential susceptibility to rearing influences: An evolutionary hypothesis and some evidence in *Origins of the social mind: Evolutionary psychology and child development,* ed. Ellis B, Bjorklund D (New York: Guildford Press, 2005), pp. 139–63.

174 *When orchid children experience a supportive, nurturing childhood:* Taylor SE, Way BM, Welch WT, et al. Early family environment, current adversity, the serotonin transporter promoter polymorphism, and depressive symptomatology. Biol Psych. 2006 Oct 1;60(7):671–76. Epub 2006 Aug 24.

174 *They do better than dandelions:* Dobbs D. The science of success, *Atlantic,* December 2009: www.theatlantic.com/magazine/archive/2009/12/the-science-of-success/7761/ (accessed March 27, 2012). In this article Dobbs describes how Stephen Suomi, PhD, a rhesus-monkey researcher who heads a set of laboratories at the National Institutes of Health's Laboratory of Comparative Ethology, was the first researcher to work with the three different forms of the serotonin gene and to conduct "gene-by-environment" studies to determine their effect. Suomi found that monkeys that carried the supposedly risky short-short gene variant and that also had nurturing mothers were better at making friends when they were young, made strong alliances as they grew older and knew how to utilize them, and handled larger group conflicts

well. They rose higher in their respective hierarchies. Despite their short serotonin gene variant they were the most successful monkeys in the troop. The implication, then, is that some brains are more plastic than others, and are therefore more affected by both positive and negative effects of supportive or unsupportive environments.

174 *what some scientists now term "DNA memories":* Hoffmann A, Spengler D. DNA memories of early social life. Neuroscience. 2012 May 7. [Epub ahead of print].

175 *Meditation studies in posttraumatic stress patients:* Hölzel BK, Carmody J, Evans KC, et al. Stress reduction correlates with structural changes in the amygdala. Soc Cogn Affect Neurosci. 2010 Mar;5(1):11–17.

Chapter Nineteen

181 *If we try to do spinal twists and balancing poses:* Broad R. *The science of yoga: The risks and rewards.* (New York: Simon & Schuster, 2012), p. 113.

181 *For instance, women who take a twelve-week:* Streeter CC, Whitfield TH, Owen L, et al. Effects of yoga versus walking on mood, anxiety, and brain GABA levels: A randomized controlled MRS study. J Altern Compl Med. 2010 Nov;16(11):1145–52.

181 *That's saying a lot:* Erickson KI, Raji CA, Lopez OL, et al. Physical activity predicts gray matter volume in late adulthood: The Cardiovascular Health Study. Neurology. 2010 Oct 19;75(16):1415–22. Barry DW, Kohrt WM. Exercise and the preservation of bone health. J Cardiopulm Rehabil Prev. 2008 May–Jun;28(3):153–62. See also "Walking: Trim your waistline, improve your health": www.mayoclinic.com/health/walking/HQ01612 (accessed March 27, 2012).

181 *They're also less likely to worry over and "catastrophize":* Carson JW, Carson KM, Jones KD, et al. A pilot randomized controlled trial of the Yoga of Awareness program in the management of fibromyalgia. Pain. 2010 Nov;151(2):530–39.

182 *They feel less fatigue and a greater sense of "emotional well-being":* Banasik J, Williams H, Haberman M, et al. Effect of Iyengar yoga practice on fatigue and diurnal salivary cortisol concentration in breast cancer survivors. J Am Acad Nurse Pract. 2011 Mar;23(3):135–42.

182 *Their pain lessens as their mood grows more positive:* Speed-Andrews AE, Stevinson C, Belanger LJ, et al. Pilot evaluation of an Iyengar Yoga program for breast cancer survivors. Cancer Nurs. 2010 Sep–Oct;33(5):369–81.

182 *Six months of yoga reduces fatigue:* Oken BS, Kishiyama S, Zajdel D, et al. Randomized controlled trial of yoga and exercise in multiple sclerosis. Neurology. 2004 Jun 8;62(11):2058–64.

182 *lessens disability, pain, and depression in adults with chronic low back pain:* Williams K, Abildso C, Steinberg L, et al. Evaluation of the effectiveness and efficacy of Iyengar yoga therapy on chronic low back pain. Spine (Phila Pa 1976). 2009 Sep 1;34(19):2066–76.

182 *lowers disease activity in patients with rheumatoid arthritis:* Badsha H, Chhabra V, Leibman C, et al. The benefits of yoga for rheumatoid arthritis: Results of a preliminary, structured 8-week program. Rheumatol Int. 2009 Oct;29(12):1417–21.

182 *and improves allergy symptoms:* Chukumnerd P, Hatthakit U, Chuaprapaisilp A. The experience of persons with allergic respiratory symptoms: Practicing yoga as a self-healing modality. Holist Nurs Pract. 2011 Mar–Apr;25(2):63–70.

182 *Cancer patients who practice yoga report:* Lin KY, Hu YT, Chang KJ, Lin HF, et al. Effects of yoga on psychological health, quality of life, and physical health of patients with cancer: A meta-analysis. Evid Based Complement Alternat Med. 2011;2011:659876. Epub 2011 Mar 9.

182 *And the thing that makes the brain decide one way or the other:* Butler D, Moseley L. *Explain pain* (Adelaide, South Australia: Noigroup Publications, 2003). In this book, Butler and Moseley discuss new findings that our level of perceived pain is based on how much the brain perceives us to be under threat. Read more on this on their blogspot: http://explainpain.blogspot.com/2007_09_23_archive.html (accessed March 28, 2012).

183 *The brain regions involved in experiencing signals of physical pain:* Macdonald G, Leary MR. Why does social exclusion hurt? The relationship between social and physical pain. Psychol Bulletin. 2005 Mar;131(2):202–23.

184 *In the study comparing those taking a three-month yoga class:* Streeter CC, Whitfield TH, Owen L, et al. Effects of yoga versus walking on mood, anxiety, and brain GABA levels: A randomized controlled MRS study. J Altern Compl Med. 2010 Nov;16(11):1145–52.

184 *Even one yoga session can significantly raise feel-good GABA:* Streeter CC, Jensen JE, Perlmutter RM, et al. Yoga Asana sessions increase brain GABA levels: A pilot study. J Altern Compl Med. 2007 May;13(4):419–26.

185 *PET scans on yoga newbies before yoga training:* Cohen DL, Wintering N, Tolles V, et al. Cerebral blood flow effects of yoga training: Preliminary evaluation of 4 cases. J Altern Compl Med. 2009 Jan;15(1):9–14.

185 *Manipulating the breath in ways that match up with a range:* Philippot P, Chapelle G, Blairy, S. Respiratory feedback in the generation of emotion. Cognition Emotion. 2002 Aug 1;16(5):605–27(23).

185 *When we combine yoga breath inhalation and retention:* Jerath R, Edry JW, Barnes VA, et al. Physiology of long pranayamic breathing: Neural respiratory elements may provide a mechanism that explains how slow deep breathing shifts the autonomic nervous system. Med Hypotheses. 2006;67(3):566–71.

186 *The vagus nerve also does something else pretty stunning:* Andersson U, Tracey KJ. Reflex principles of immunological homeostasis. Annu Rev Immunol. 2012 Apr 23;30:313–35.

187 *And this, in turn, causes a slowing of brain wave activity:* Streeter CC, Gerbarg PL, Saper RB, et al. Effects of yoga on the autonomic nervous system, gamma-aminobutyric-acid, and allostasis in epilepsy, depression, and post-traumatic stress disorder. Med Hypotheses. 2012 Feb 24. [Epub ahead of print]. Brown RP, Gerbarg PL. Yoga breathing, meditation, and longevity. Ann N Y Acad Sci. 2009 Aug;1172:54–62.

187 *This long-term physiological switch toward "parasympathetic dominance":* Curtis K, Osadchuk A, Katz J, et al. An eight-week yoga intervention is associated with improvements in pain, psychological functioning and mindfulness, and changes in cortisol levels in women with fibromyalgia. J Pain Res. 2011;4:189–201.

189 *The more neural stem cells divide, the more neurogenesis you undergo:* Reynolds G. Phys ed: Your brain on exercise, *New York Times* blog, "Well": http://well.blogs.nytimes.com/2010/07/07/your-brain-on-exercise/ (accessed March 27, 2012).

189 *Exercise profoundly stimulates the production of Noggin:* van Praag H, Shubert T, Zhao C, et al. Exercise enhances learning and hippocampal neurogenesis in aged mice. J Neurosci. 2005 Sep 21;25(38):8680–85. Farmer J, Zhao X, van Praag H, et al. Effects of voluntary exercise on synaptic plasticity and gene expression in the dentate gyrus of adult male Sprague-Dawley rats in vivo. Neuroscience. 2004;124(1):71–79.

189 *There are clear links that suggest that physical activity in general:* Schloesser RJ, Lehmann M, Martinowich K, et al. Environmental enrichment requires adult neurogenesis to facilitate the recovery from psychosocial stress. Mol Psychiatry. 2010 Dec;15(12):1152–63. In this study conducted at the Source Laboratory of Molecular Pathophysiology at the

National Institute of Mental Health (NIMH), researchers divided mice into two groups: aggressive alpha mice and smaller, less assertive mice. They put the smaller mice into cages with the more aggressive rodents, leaving only a clear partition between them. Occasionally they removed the partition, and restrained the larger mouse from harming the smaller one, that had nowhere to go. The runtlike mice were, however, treated differently prior to the study. One group of smaller mice was allowed to exercise on running wheels and explore in tubes for several weeks before the experiment; the punier mice were not. After two weeks of being exposed to the hostile mice, the group that had been allowed to exercise before their stressful experience exhibited "stress-resistant" behavior, say researchers. The other mice, who hadn't had two weeks of exercise before meeting their scary roommate, exhibited distinct signs of severe anxiety and depression. Even when they were taken out of their cages and introduced to other sources of stress they hid in dark corners. They froze with fear. It turns out that the stress-resistant mice had more neurons firing in the area of the brain known as the medial prefrontal cortex, an area of the brain involved in emotional processing. Researchers point out that this change toward a healthier stress response was significant even when the smaller mice were exposed to quite moderate levels of exercise.

189 *In a recent evaluation of a number of studies that show physical activity:* Ernst C, Olson AK, Pinel JP, et al. Antidepressant effects of exercise: Evidence for an adult-neurogenesis hypothesis? J Psychiatry Neurosci. 2006 Mar;31(2):84–92.

190 *And experts believe that yoga in particular may facilitate:* Simpkins AM, Simpkins CA. *Meditation and yoga in psychotherapy: Techniques for clinical practice* (Hoboken, NJ: John Wiley & Sons, 2011), p. 32.

190 *In animal studies, exercise increases the number of stem cells:* Shefer G, Rauner G, Yablonka-Reuveni Z, et al. Reduced satellite cell numbers and myogenic capacity in aging can be alleviated by endurance exercise. PLoS One. 2010 Oct 12;5(10):e13307.

190 *In one humorous study, well-exercised mice didn't undergo the changes in fur:* Safdar A, Bourgeois JM, Ogborn DI, et al. Endurance exercise rescues progeroid aging and induces systemic mitochondrial rejuvenation in mtDNA mutator mice. Proc Natl Acad Sci U S A. 2011 Mar 8;108(10):4135–40.

190 *Women under stress who exercise have longer telomeres:* Puterman E, Lin J, Blackburn E, et al. The power of exercise: Buffering the effect of chronic stress on telomere length. PLoS One. 2010 May 26;5(5):e10837.

190 *It helps to know, too, that just fifteen minutes of physical activity:* Wen CP, Wai JP, Tsai MK, et al. Minimum amount of physical activity for reduced mortality and extended life expectancy: A prospective cohort study. Lancet. 2011 Oct 1;378(9798):1244–53.

190 *Being active reduces frequency and severity of colds:* Nieman DC, Henson DA, Austin MD, et al. Upper respiratory tract infection is reduced in physically fit and active adults.Br J Sports Med. 2011 Sep;45(12):987–92.

190 *and our risk of Alzheimer's:* Stranahan AM, Martin B, Maudsley S. Anti-inflammatory effects of physical activity in relationship to improved cognitive status in humans and mouse models of Alzheimer's disease. Curr Alzheimer Res. 2012 Jan 1;9(1):86–92.

Chapter Twenty

195 *proving to be remarkably helpful in patients suffering from back pain:* Büssing A, Ostermann T, Lüdtke R, et al. Effects of yoga interventions on pain and pain-associated disability: A meta-analysis. J Pain. 2012 Jan;13(1):1–9.

Chapter Twenty-two

203 *We're plunking ourselves down more than ever:* Clark N. Sedentary athletes: Sitting and weighting, American College of Sports Medicine, *Fit Society Newsletter,* Winter 2009–2010. In this article Clark discusses a talk given by Neville Owen, PhD, speaker at the American College of Sports Medicine's Annual Meeting in May 2009, in which he shares data showing that the average American sits 9.3 hours a day: www.sportsmd.com/SportsMD_Articles/id/382/n/sedentary_athletes_sitting_and_weighting.aspx (accessed March 28, 2012). See also Dunstan DW, Owen N. New exercise prescription: Don't just sit there: Stand up and move more, more often: Comment on "sitting time and all-cause mortality risk in 222,497 Australian adults." Arch Intern Med. 2012 Mar 26;172(6):500–501.

203 *A woman who sits just six hours a day:* Patel AV, Bernstein L, Deka A, et al. Leisure time spent sitting in relation to total mortality in a prospective cohort of US adults. Am J Epidemiol. 2010 Aug 15;172(4):419–29. Epub 2010 Jul 22.

203 *People who sit for most of the day are 54 percent:* Katzmarzyk PT, Church TS, Craig CL, et al. Sitting time and mortality from all causes, cardiovascular disease, and cancer. Med Sci Sports Exerc. 2009 May;41(5):998–1005.

203 *People who sit and watch TV for three hours:* In 2011, the trade group for individuals involved in desk jobs related to medical billing and coding put out an infographic that gathered together a number of government statistics to show the damaging effects of sitting for those in their largely sedentary industry. This infographic can be found at www.medicalbillingandcoding.org/sitting-kills/ (accessed March 28, 2012). One recent study found that compared to people who spend fewer than two hours each day on screen-based entertainment like watching TV, using the computer, or playing video games, those who devote more than four hours to screen time a day are more than twice as likely to have a major cardiac event that involves hospitalization, death, or both: Stamatakis E, Hamer M, Dunstan DW. Screen-based entertainment time, all-cause mortality, and cardiovascular events: Population-based study with ongoing mortality and hospital events follow-up. J Am Coll Cardiol. 2011 Jan 18;57(3):292–99. For more information on this discussion on sedentary behavior see also: Thorp AA, Owen N, Neuhaus M, et al. Sedentary behaviors and subsequent health outcomes in adults a systematic review of longitudinal studies, 1996–2011. Am J Prev Med. 2011 Aug;41(2):207–15. Salmon J, Tremblay MS, Marshall SJ, et al. Health risks, correlates, and interventions to reduce sedentary behavior in young people. Am J Prev Med. 2011 Aug;41(2):197–206. Owen N, Healy GN, Matthews CE, et al. Too much sitting: The population health science of sedentary behavior. Exerc Sport Sci Rev. 2010 Jul;38(3):105–13. Gardiner PA, Healy GN, Eakin EG, et al. Associations between television viewing time and overall sitting time with the metabolic syndrome in older men and women: The Australian Diabetes, Obesity and Lifestyle Study. J Am Geriatr Soc. 2011 May;59(5):788–96. Bauman A, Ainsworth BE, Sallis JF, et al. The descriptive epidemiology of sitting a 20-country comparison using the International Physical Activity Questionnaire (IPAQ). Am J Prev Med. 2011 Aug;41(2):228–35.

203 *And each extra hour of TV you watch adds up to an 11 percent*: Bauman A, Ainsworth BE, Sallis JF, et al. Television viewing time and mortality: The Australian Diabetes, Obesity and Lifestyle Study (AusDiab). Circulation. 2010 Jan 26;121(3):384–91.

203 *The shocker is that these differences are even seen:* www.medicalbillingandcoding.org/sitting-kills/ (accessed March 28, 2012).

204 *Our level of C-reactive protein:* Healy GN, Matthews CE, Dunstan DW, et al. Sed-

entary time and cardio-metabolic biomarkers in US adults: NHANES 2003–06. Eur Heart J. 2011 Mar;32(5):590–97.

204 *When a certain enzyme, called lipoprotein lipase (LPL):* Vlahos J. Is sitting a lethal activity? *New York Times Magazine*, April 14, 2011. This can also be viewed online at: www.nytimes.com/2011/04/17/magazine/mag-17sitting-t.html?_r=1 (accessed March 28, 2012).

204 *for regulating glucose and fat begin to shut down:* Ekblom-Bak E, Hellénius ML, Ekblom B. Are we facing a new paradigm of inactivity physiology? Br J Sports Med. 2010 Sep;44(12):834–35.

211 *I like knowing that when we practice these and other weight-bearing yoga:* Phoosuwan M, Kritpet T, Yuktanandana P. The effects of weight bearing yoga training on the bone resorption markers of the postmenopausal women. J Med Assoc Thai. 2009 Sep;92(Suppl 5):S102–S108.

Chapter Twenty-three

212 *For the first few minutes we do simple exercises:* In addition to learning laughter yoga with Mira Tessman, I also took a local community laughter yoga class with Deb Donofrio, in Baltimore, Maryland. To find out more you can reach Deb at yoga forchildren@comcast.net.

213 *"A stress lifted from my soul. It lifted from my body":* Raffi Khatchadourian reports on this vignette in his article, The laughing guru: Madan Kataria's prescription for total well-being, *New Yorker*, August 30, 2010, p. 58.

213 *Around the globe we all laugh in the same pattern:* Robert R. Provine, *Laughter: A scientific investigation* (New York: Viking, 2000). See also: To scientists, laughter is no joke, at *CBS News*, which discusses the work of neuroscientist Robert Provine and his studies on the commonality of laughter: www.cbsnews.com/stories/2010/03/31/tech/main6350777.shtml (accessed March 28, 2012).

214 *protecting against heart disease:* Miller M, Fry WF. The effect of mirthful laughter on the human cardiovascular system. Med Hypotheses. 2009 Nov;73(5):636–39. Sugawara J, Tarumi T, Tanaka H. Effect of mirthful laughter on vascular function. Am J Cardiol. 2010 Sep 15;106(6):856–59.

214 *lowering inflammation in patients with diabetes:* Tan SA, Tan LG, Lukman ST, et al. Humor, as an adjunct therapy in cardiac rehabilitation, attenuates catecholamines and myocardial infarction recurrence. Adv Mind Body Med. 2007 Winter;22(3–4):8–12.

214 *combating depression:* Shahidi M, Mojtahed A, Modabbernia A, et al. Laughter yoga versus group exercise program in elderly depressed women: A randomized controlled trial. Int J Geriatr Psych. 2011 Mar;26(3):322–27.

214 *protecting the immune system:* Berk LS, Felten DL, Tan SA, et al. Modulation of neuroimmune parameters during the eustress of humor-associated mirthful laughter. Altern Ther Health Med. 2001 Mar;7(2):62–72, 74–76.

214 *and improving the quality of life for breast cancer survivors:* Cho EA, Oh HE. Effects of laughter therapy on depression, quality of life, resilience and immune responses in breast cancer survivors. J Korean Acad Nurs. 2011 Jun;41(3):285–93.

214 *caused arteries to restrict 30 to 50 percent:* Miller M, Mangano C, Park Y, et al. Impact of cinematic viewing on endothelial function. Heart. 2006 February;92(2):261–62.

214 *If we merely think about watching a humorous video:* Berk LS. Studying the biology of hope: An interview with Lee S. Berk, DrPH, MPH. Interview by Sheldon Lewis. Adv Mind Body Med. 2007 Summer;22(2):28–31.

214 *Howling, just for the record:* Neuhoff CC, Schaefer C. Effects of laughing, smiling, and howling on mood. Psychol Rep. 2002 Dec;91(3 Pt 2):1079–80.
216 *In reality, our red blood cells:* Broad R. *The science of yoga: The risks and rewards* (New York: Simon & Schuster 2012), 84–87.

Chapter Twenty-four

219 *The Mayo Clinic recently reported that acupuncture:* Martin DP, Sletten CD, Williams BA, et al. Improvement in fibromyalgia symptoms with acupuncture: Results of a randomized controlled trial. Mayo Clin Proc. 2006 Jun;81(6):749–57.
219 *For women with PCOS:* Raja-Khan N, Stener-Victorin E, Wu X, et al. The physiological basis of complementary and alternative medicines for polycystic ovary syndrome. Am J Physiol Endocrinol Metab. 2011 Jul;301(1):E1–E10.
219 *the strong eye to help strengthen the weak one:* Zhao J, Lam DS, Chen LJ, et al. Randomized controlled trial of patching vs acupuncture for anisometropic amblyopia in children aged 7 to 12 years. Arch Ophthalmol. 2010 Dec;128(12):1510–17.
220 *reducing the degree of pain we actually feel:* Radiological Society of North America. Acupuncture changes brain's perception and processing of pain, researchers find. *ScienceDaily*, November 30, 2010: www.sciencedaily.com/releases/2010/11/101130 100357.htm (accessed March 28, 2012). These findings were presented at the annual meeting of the Radiological Society of North America (RSNA) in November 2010. The study was conducted by Nina Theysohn, MD, from the Department of Diagnostic and Interventional Radiology and Neuroradiology at University Hospital in Essen, Germany.
220 *Similarly, when researchers press very warm heat:* Shukla S, Torossian A, Duann JR, et al. The analgesic effect of electroacupuncture on acute thermal pain perception—a central neural correlate study with fMRI. Mol Pain. 2011 Jun 7;7:45.
220 *dependable treatment for lower back pain:* Schmitt H, Zhao JQ, Brocai DR, et al. Acupuncture treatment of low back pain. Schmerz. 2001 Feb;15(1).33 37
220 *When activated, these receptors:* Harris RE, Zubieta JK, Scott DJ, et al. Traditional Chinese acupuncture and placebo (sham) acupuncture are differentiated by their effects on mu-opioid receptors (MORs). Neuroimage. 2009 Sep;47(3):1077–85.
221 *Mu-opioid receptors regulate the function:* Zubieta JK, Ketter TA, Bueller JA, et al. Regulation of human affective responses by anterior cingulate and limbic mu-opioid neurotransmission. Arch Gen Psychiatry. 2003 Nov;60(11):1145–53.
221 *Injected mice given acupuncture had fewer pain:* Goldman N, Chen M, Fujita T, et al. Adenosine A1 receptors mediate local anti-nociceptive effects of acupuncture. Nat Neurosci. 2010 Jul;13(7):883–88.
221 *as medication for relieving nausea:* El-Deeb AM, Ahmady MS. Effect of acupuncture on nausea and/or vomiting during and after cesarean section in comparison with ondansetron. J Anesth. 2011 Oct;25(5):698–703.
222 *a sham placebo acupuncture treatment:* Enblom A, Johnsson A, Hammar M, et al. Acupuncture compared with placebo acupuncture in radiotherapy-induced nausea—a randomized controlled study. Ann Oncol. 2011 Sep 23. [Epub ahead of print]
222 *Both the patients who received genuine and sham:* Enblom A, Lekander M, Hammar M, et al. Getting the grip on nonspecific treatment effects: Emesis in patients randomized to acupuncture or sham compared to patients receiving standard care. PLoS One. 2011 Mar 23;6(3):e14766.
222 *these same biochemical changes in our brain:* Lai X, Zhang G, Huang Y, et al. A cerebral functional imaging study by positron emission tomography in healthy volun-

teers receiving true or sham acupuncture needling. Neurosci Lett. 2009 Mar 13;452(2):194–99. Harris RE, Zubieta JK, Scott DJ, et al. Traditional Chinese acupuncture and placebo (sham) acupuncture are differentiated by their effects on mu-opioid receptors (MORs). Neuroimage. 2009 Sep;47(3):1077–85. Hui KK, Liu J, Makris N, Gollub RL, et al. Acupuncture modulates the limbic system and subcortical gray structures of the human brain: Evidence from fMRI studies in normal subjects. Hum Brain Mapp. 2000;9(1):13–25. Napadow V, Kettner N, Liu J, et al. Hypothalamus and amygdala response to acupuncture stimuli in carpal tunnel syndrome. Pain. 2007 August;130(3):254–66. Molassiotis A, Sylt P, Diggins H. The management of cancer-related fatigue after chemotherapy with acupuncture and acupressure: A randomised controlled trial. Complement Ther Med. 2007 Dec;15(4):228–37.

222 *with the temporary relief of pain:* Hui KK, Liu J, Makris N, et al. Acupuncture modulates the limbic system and subcortical gray structures of the human brain: Evidence from fMRI studies in normal subjects. Hum Brain Mapp. 2000;9(1):13–25.

223 *Acupressure, we know, is a well-proven*: Robinson N, Lorenc A, Liao X. The evidence for Shiatsu: A systematic review of Shiatsu and acupressure. BMC Compl Altern Med. 2011 Oct 7;11(1):88.

223 *physical stressors that may influence his or her pain and health:* Karst M. Comment on "Acupuncture: Does it alleviate pain and are there serious risks? A review of reviews" Ernst et al. [Pain 2011;152:755–64]. Pain. 2011 Sep;152(9):2181; author reply 2184–86.

224 *your fingers over money relieves chronic pain:* Zhou X, Vohs KD, Baumeister RF. The symbolic power of money: Reminders of money alter social distress and physical pain. Psychol Sci. 2009 Jun;20(6):700–706. You can read about this study at: www.livescience.com/health/090724-money-pain.html (accessed March 28, 2012).

224 *or the expectation of a good, pain-free outcome:* Radiological Society of North America. Acupuncture changes brain's perception and processing of pain, researchers find. *ScienceDaily*, November 30, 2010: www.sciencedaily.com/releases/2010/11/101130100357.htm (accessed March 28, 2012). These findings were presented at the annual meeting of the Radiological Society of North America (RSNA) in November 2010. The study was conducted by Nina Theysohn, MD, from the Department of Diagnostic and Interventional Radiology and Neuroradiology at University Hospital in Essen, Germany.

Index